The Magic of Fat Loss

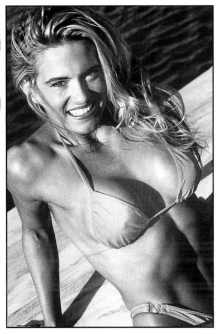

Lose Fat and Double Your Energy For Life!

By Robert Kennedy
and Dwayne Hines II

D1370546

Published by MuscleMag International
5775 McLaughlin Road
Mississauga, ON Canada
L5R 3P7

Designed by Jackie Kydyk

Canadian Cataloguing in Publication Data

Kennedy, Robert, 1938-
   The magic of fat loss: lose fat and double your
energy for life!

Includes bibliographical references and index.

   1. Reducing exercises. I. Hines, Dwayne, 1961-
II. Title.

RA781.6.K46   1997   646.7'5   C97-900858-1

ISBN 1-55210-006-5

10 9 8 7 6 5 4 3 Pbk

Distributed in Canada by
CANBOOK Distribution Services
1220 Nicholson Road
Newmarket, ON
L3Y 7V1
1-800-399-6858

Distributed in the United States by
BookWorld Services
1933 Whitfield Park Loop
Sarasota, FL 34243

Printed in Canada

Dedicated to Bill Scott and Heather
Special note of thanks to Janet for research help.

Table of Contents

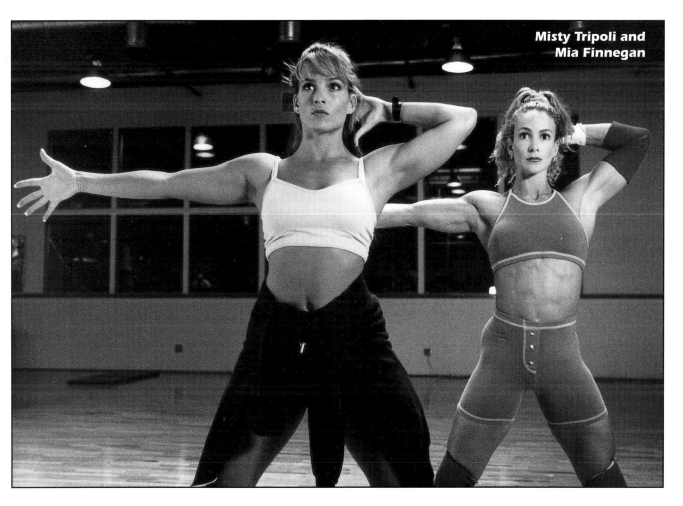

Misty Tripoli and
Mia Finnegan

Lose Fat and Double Your Energy For Life! – **THE MAGIC OF FAT LOSS**

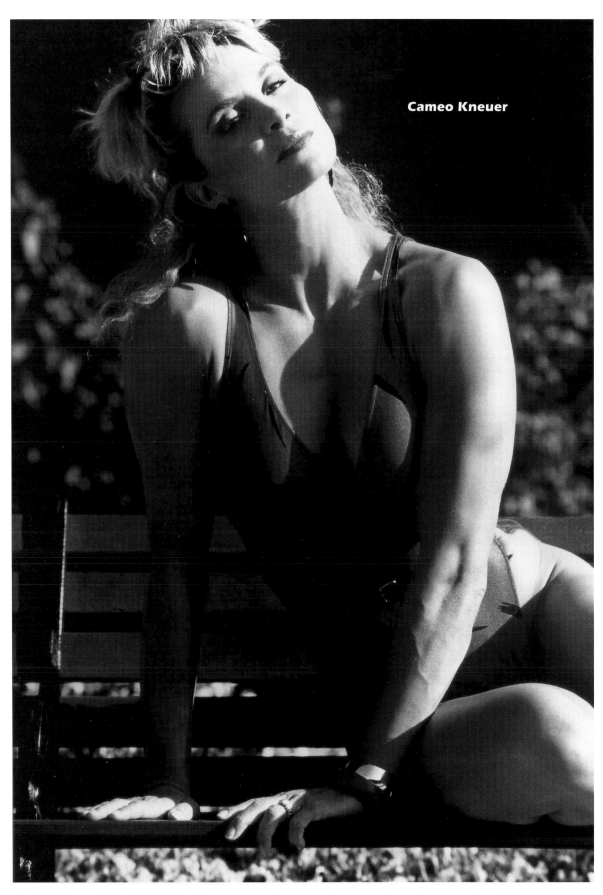

Cameo Kneuer

CHAPTER ONE

Aerobics, Metabolism and a Fit Physique

Fat is the archnemesis of anyone – at least of any woman who has real concerns about the appearance of her physique and the quality of her health. Fat is hated by the general public (for example, look at the trim physiques of the fashion models), but is hated even more by the fitness community. Fat hides those toned muscles that are the result of all the precious time and tremendous effort in the gym. Fat takes the definite edge off the body and gives it a round and bloated appearance. Fat has been the downfall of many a hopeful fitness star. And fat is not a pushover when it comes to these weight wars – it is a very tough enemy to beat. For instance, the bodybuilding community strives to have the least bodyfat, yet even this group has a tough go with fighting fat. Many fitness stars try to use

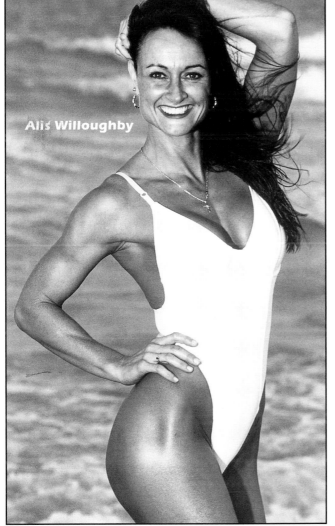

Alis Willoughby

extreme diets and certain food fads to knock out fat. Despite all of the good intentions, however, an estimated 90 percent of people who go on a diet will regain all or most of the weight they lose.[1] That is because fat is deceiving – it hides behind delicious, tempting covers. It creates deep food cravings that cause a person to do almost anything to fulfill them. And overcoming that intense food craving, that desire for another tasty meal, is not easy. Many physique trainers note that getting rid of excess bodyweight is the toughest thing for a person to do – and most people are not successful at it. This continual struggle against fat is just as tough, and perhaps even more so, for a person trying to stay in shape than for the average citizen. Consider the following story about a physique competitor:

"Three days before the 1988 USA Bodybuilding Championships, I found Stoney at the grocery store at midnight with an entire cart full of food. A few months later, just before the Nationals, he disappeared again. This time, I found him at 2:00 a.m. parked next to the drive thru at Jolly Pirate Donuts. He was sitting in the car completely covered in sugar from at least three-dozen donuts, and he was working on another three dozen or so that were sitting on the passenger seat."[2]

It is not easy to beat the "fat monster," especially when there are so many fantastic and delicious foods around. Ice cream, muffins, donuts, pizza, chocolate cake, cream pie – all taste as good as ever. Just because you want to stay in shape does not mean the "forbidden food" tastes any less delicious. Usually it tastes even better because it is forbidden. You can see everyone else having the tasty food, but you can't have it. This can lead to heavy-duty temptation and sometimes a large binge by the dieting person. Stoney is not the only example of this. For reference sake, here is another example:

"Quite a few years ago a *big*-name bodybuilder came to town to give a lecture… the first thing I noticed was that he didn't eat like he stated in the magazines. You know the training articles with those pictures where they sit down to eat in posing trunks and only have a small piece of broiled fish and a glass of tea. He actually ate like a pig, devouring everything in sight like pizza, ice cream, pancakes, etc."[3]

Fat hides behind many different delicious, tempting covers.

It is no myth: Those who are into fitness as a lifestyle are just as susceptible to tasty and nasty fatty foods as anyone else. It takes iron discipline and a deep commitment to win the food game and master your physique. Not many are able to do it. Fat often wins the war. Again, consider the plight of those most serious about low bodyfat levels, the bodybuilders. A large number of physique stars are substantially overweight during the off-season. That is why the photo shoots for the magazines are done right before or after a competition – many of the bodybuilders are too fat to have their picture taken during the rest of the year. Some have even been known to gain *double-digit* poundage the week or two after a big contest. But most bodybuilders, and those interested in a fit physique do not give in to fat that easily. Many try to quell this "fat" rebellion and fight back by going on an even tougher diet. A tough diet is not always enough, and you can take dieting only so far. In order to beat fat, more firepower is needed. One of the best ways to beat fat is to not rely totally on the diet. A better plan is

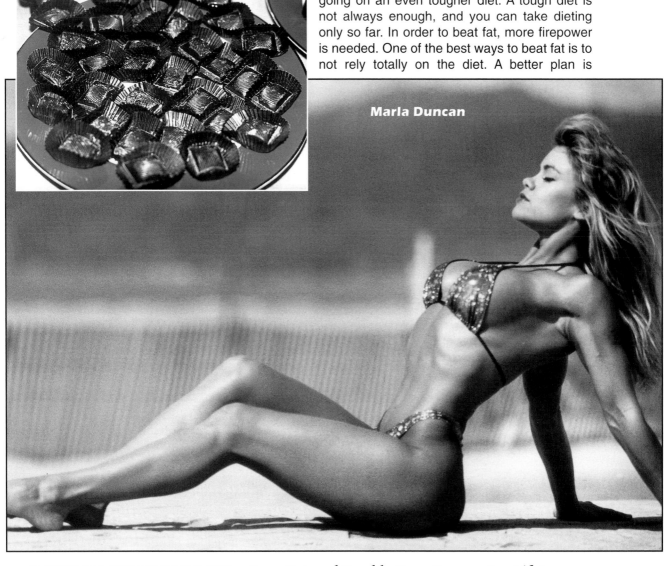

Marla Duncan

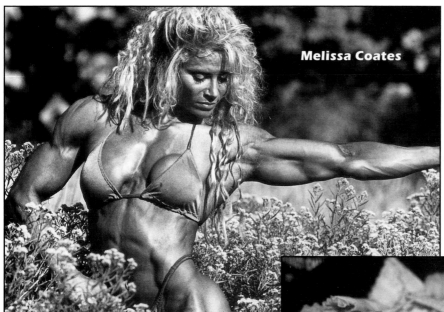

Melissa Coates

overcome the body's fat stores. A single-pronged attack on fat (diet alone) is not nearly enough to substantially reduce fat – a strong triple-combination punch is necessary. This effective and efficient combination is diet, aerobic exercise, and weight training working together. Diet restricts the intake of fat for the body, and aerobic

When dieting, forbidden food usually begins to taste better than it normally would.

through a three-pronged attack. The actions necessary to "triple team" fat are diet, aerobic exercise and weight training. These three, acting together, make a powerful front to fight fat.

> ## Aerobic exercise, if done properly, uses fat for fuel.

Diet

Your diet is a crucial element in controlling the level of bodyfat that you carry. Getting the diet right is not as easy as everyone thinks. Everyone has a diet – but not everyone's diet is good. The best diet supplies you with all of the necessary nutrients without supplying you with too much of some element. The amounts and combinations of certain foods are important, as is timing. In fact, timing of your eating habits is vital. For more information on diet check out the nutrition section at your local bookstore.

Aerobic Action

Aerobic exercise is an awesome tool in the fight against fat because aerobic exercise, if done properly, uses fat for fuel. This assists greatly in the triple-team effort that is necessary to

exercise uses any fat that does get by the diet as fuel. Weight training further burns off any accumulated fat. Most people, especially those who are in tune to fitness, are well-versed in restricting the diet to avoid fat and sugar (which, taken in excess, also causes the body to become fatter). They know, however, that aerobic action is too vital to overlook.

Muscular Conditioning

There is another factor in looking great that requires more than just aerobics, and it's muscular training. A body that is weight trained has better shape than if it is not weight trained. Also when a body has more muscle, it burns off more fat throughout the day. So weight training has a double-positive effect. One of the most famous physique stars ever, Rachel McLish, noted the benefits of shaping the body through weight training:

"As beneficial as aerobic exercise is, it's not enough to reshape your body to the perfect proportions you'd like to see reflected in your

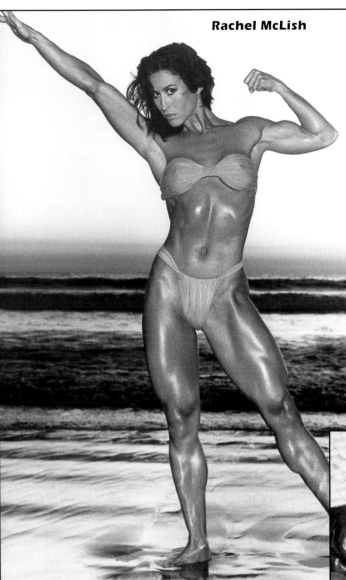

Rachel McLish

Focused Training

This book focuses on using the tools of aerobic and muscular exercise for getting rid of the fat you want to get rid of. Aerobic exercise is a very productive way to strip the fat off the physique, and muscular exercise hypes the metabolic rate for further fat reduction. This approach works particularly well for the woman who is concerned with her physique and her special training needs.

Not every aerobic exercise is a good one though. For instance, running is a vigorous conditioner for the body's largest and most powerful muscles, especially the heart. Studies have shown repeatedly that running significantly improves cardiovascular fitness for almost everyone, including children and older people. Runners show a lower percentage of overall bodyfat than any other group (including competitive cyclists, rowers, swimmers, etc.).[5] Many fitness authorities point to the fact that running is the quickest way to get rid of fat. If someone wants to lose weight rapidly, they are often advised to "start running."

mirror. To do that you've got to do more than burn off fat; you've got to build and shape your muscles. It may be satisfying to see fat dropping off your frame, but in the long run wouldn't you rather build curves and firm flesh where you want it rather than just settle for a somewhat thinner shapelessness?"[4]

By building up some muscle shape and tone, you not only add curves and firm flesh in the right areas, as Rachel notes, but you also set your metabolism higher, which causes you to burn off more bodyfat consistently. The increase in muscle will boost your metabolism, and you will increase the amount of calories that your body uses. This is the basic reason an active person stays trimmer on more calories than a sedentary person does on fewer calories.

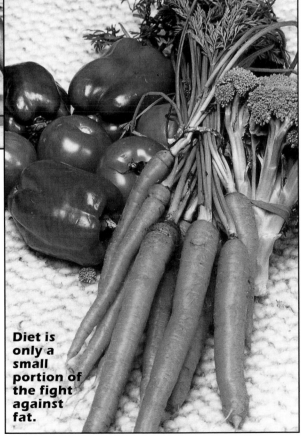

Diet is only a small portion of the fight against fat.

Before you take up running, though, there are a couple of other points to consider including that some of the very factors that make running such a vigorous conditioner can also cause injuries. For instance, the force which is generated between your foot and the ground can amount to up to 2.8 times your bodyweight during fast running and 5.5 times your bodyweight during sprinting. Foot-strike impact can amount to a force of 30 Gs. Despite the body's shock-absorbing capabilities, most runners are well aware that they are not immune to injuries. In a survey of entrants in a 10-kilometer road race in New York City, researchers found that 46.6 percent of the respondents had sustained a running injury within the previous two years. [6]

Injuries are a big problem and should be avoided at all cost. An injury can really set a training program back. Time is a superprecious commodity for almost every woman who is serious about reshaping her physique, and such a person cannot afford to lose training time to an injury caused by an aerobic workout. Unfortunately, a person can easily injure the lower body while running, especially if the running is performed on a regular basis and on a hard surface.

Injuries are not the only negative consideration when it comes to the use of running as the prime aerobic exercise. The other is the big taboo, overtraining. Many personal trainers point out that running causes the body to quickly go into a state of overtraining, throwing the body into a semishock condition. This makes muscle-tone gains come to a screeching halt, and

Running too much on a regular basis can cause lower-body injuries and also a state of overtraining.

allows fat accumulation or sloppy muscle tone to re-occur in a quirky action of nature. Running on a regular basis is said to inhibit further muscular gains and, if at a very intense level, running can cut into previous muscle-tone gains. This is a situation the person concerned about reshaping the physique wants to totally avoid.

When a person runs hard, the body's recuperation process is primarily used for handling the running routine and adapting the body to that strenuous work instead of on building the body up and reshaping the physique. The same is true for the use of the body's energy stores, which are so vital to successful body shaping. Running long and hard on a regular basis really dips into the body's reserves, leaving little or nothing for the muscles to be replenished with,

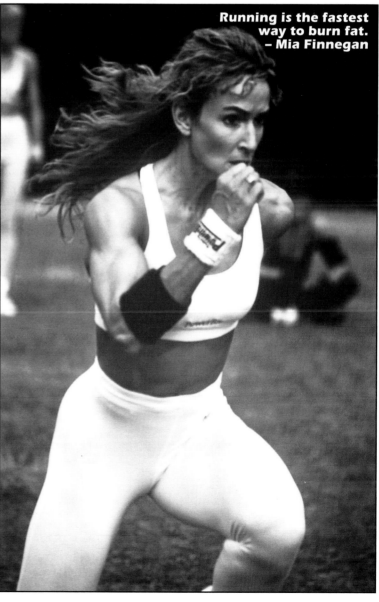

Running is the fastest way to burn fat.
– Mia Finnegan

and little or nothing for the various upcoming workouts. For these primary reasons, personal trainers, for the most part, advise their clientele to strictly avoid too much running, especially when on a program for reshaping the physique through muscle gains. A person may be able to get away with one run a week or maybe even two shorter runs, but going too far beyond this range can cause problems.

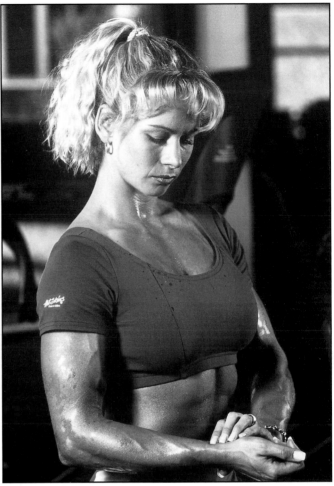

Dr. Christine Lydon monitors the intensity of her workouts to avoid overtraining.

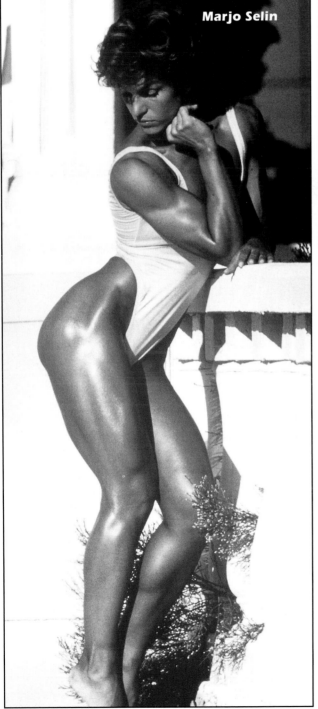

Marjo Selin

Not every aerobic exercise is going to work for every woman who wishes to reshape her physique. What works for the general public in the aerobic arena will not necessarily work well for the woman who wants to take control of the shape of her body, because there are certain needs which must be met when shaping the physique. You do not necessarily want to burn off all your bodyfat and build no muscle. This depleted state causes you to look like a skinny, sickly scarecrow. To have an attractive physique, a certain amount of muscle is necessary. Fat loss must work hand in hand with some muscle gains. To accomplish this your body has certain specific needs. These needs are:
• an aerobic exercise that will burn off fat without throwing the body into a state of overtraining.
• an aerobic exercise that will not have a tendency to cause injuries – even if they are just small, nagging ones.

Running too long and hard can cut into your muscular gains by depleting your energy reserves.

These two items must be given attention and priority when considering an aerobic routine for reshaping your physique. Ignoring these crucial factors can really throw off your physique-training program.

Not All Aerobic Exercises Are Created Equal!

Certain aerobic exercises will work well for the woman trying to reshape her physique, and others will not work so great. When it comes to the viewpoint of successfully reshaping the body on all fronts (fat loss and increased muscle tone), not all aerobic exercises are equal. Some aerobic exercises, such as running, cause more problems than they are worth. This book is going to spotlight the best of the aerobic exercises for the very specific needs of those interested in reshaping the body with the goal of less fat and more muscle tone.

Most of the better aerobic exercises have been discovered through trial and error. You can avoid the long search for the best body-shaping aerobics by using what has been discovered to your training advantage. Champion physique star Porter Cottrell is one example of a person who found the best aerobic exercises for his training through trial and error. He notes:

"In the past, my aerobic activity consisted of simply getting on a bike and spinning my wheels. I wasn't really elevating my heart rate this way! When performing aerobic activity it is important that you make sure you've elevated your heart rate to 70 percent of your maximum. I can't underscore this enough. So many people

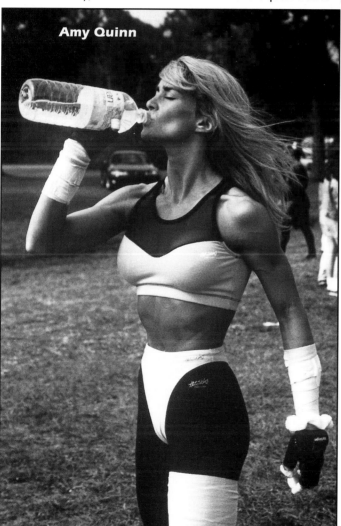

Amy Quinn

Not every aerobic exercise will work for the woman trying to reshape her physique. There are specific needs when it comes to aerobic training.

who engage in aerobic activity for the purpose of dropping bodyfat don't do this and, as a result, are just spinning their wheels. If your goal is to build solid muscle, lose bodyfat, or both you have to keep your metabolism primed. In this respect, I've learned that my body responds best to two forms of aerobic exercise: the stair stepper and fast walking. These are the two best exercises for me to burn bodyfat."[7] Porter discovered the combination of exercises which allowed him to get into razor-sharp contest

To successfully burn fat your body needs recuperation and replenishment as much as it needs stimulation and intensity.

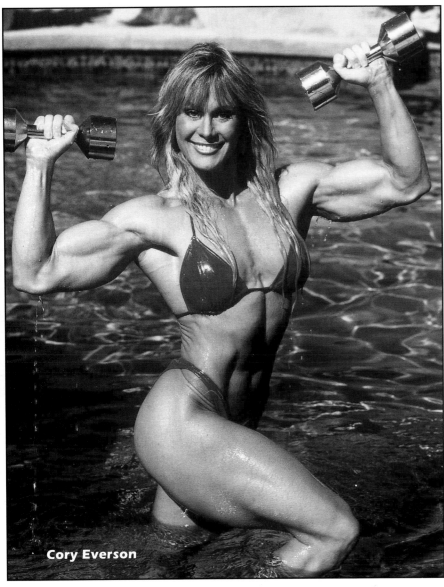

Cory Everson

to use the aerobic exercise that does not cause the loss. Choosing the right aerobic exercise is important for the ultimate shaping of your physique.

Low-impact Exercise

Another of the primary necessities in a good aerobic exercise for those who want to reshape their physique is that the exercise in question be a low-impact exercise. A low-impact exercise is one in which the body structure is not jolted too strongly during the performance of the exercise. High-impact exercises really shock the body and a continual pounding on the body can cause injury. Running and jumping rope are examples of high-impact exercises, especially when performed on a solid surface like concrete. The reason a person should avoid the high-impact exercises is obvious – the more time spent on them, the more chance there is of becoming injured with either a small, nagging injury or a more major one. Injuries short-circuit training time, forcing you to miss the time you should be spending on muscle toning. This program recommends

It is crucial to know which aerobic exercises work well for shaping the body and which do not work so well.

condition without sacrificing muscle by experimenting with different routines. Consider his advice, along with that of other physique competitors, to determine what will work for you.

If a certain aerobic exercise causes a loss in muscle tone (due to overtraining or the shock effect of too much stimulation), that exercise needs to be replaced by one that does not cause a lot of muscle loss for obvious reasons. If two aerobic exercises can be used for burning off bodyfat and one of the two causes significant muscle loss while the other does not, it is wise

using low-impact exercises that keep the body healthy and in the gym.

The aerobic exercises that will provide the most successful results are those which allow for a lean condition without sacrificing muscle tone.

20-minute Mark

A crucial element for an effective aerobic exercise is that it last long enough to have a fat-burning effect. An exercise that does not last this long is not going to burn off bodyfat, and will consume glycogen instead of fat for fuel. In order for your body to switch from using glycogen for fuel to using fat for fuel you will need to exercise nonstop for longer than 20 minutes. It is roughly at the 20-minute mark (this

High-impact aerobic exercises should be avoided for those wishing to attain long-term results.

point may vary somewhat) where the body starts to draw upon fat reserves for fuel. If you are accustomed to dashing off a quick mile, or spending a hurried 10 minutes on the stair stepper, or taking a few laps in the pool, you have really accomplished nothing at all except burn glycogen. If you quit exercising after 10 to 20 minutes, you will not have touched on getting at your fat stores. So in order to use fat for fuel, you need to make your aerobic exercise last for longer than 20 minutes. Some people make the mistake of just going up to the 20-minute mark. But this 20-minute mark is only the starting point, a longer exercise session is actually needed if you want to strip the fat off your physique. This is an important piece of knowledge that you will want to take advantage of if you hope to become trimmer and obtain that great ultratoned look. The ladies who have conquered their physique through cardiovascular work use a workout that lasts for longer than 20 minutes. For example, fitness star Marla Duncan uses a 35- to 45-minute cardiovascular workout several times a week.[8] Cameo Kneuer suggests getting in at least 20 to 30 minutes of cardio/aerobic work several times a week.[9] Tatiana Anderson performs 45 minutes of aerobic work a day.[10] Dayna Albrecht utilizes aerobics for daily 30-minute sessions.[11] Nikki Fuller uses much more than 45 minutes when training for a physique competition.[12] Lisa Smith, 1995 Ms. Louisiana, uses a 30-minute workout or more.[13] Notice that these ladies go beyond 20 minutes. When you work out, make certain

to focus on going *past* 20 minutes of aerobic exercise. You have to go beyond 20 minutes to get the best benefits from your aerobic session. Of course, at first you will want to work your way up to longer workouts, but once you have put down an aerobic-training foundation, you can then move on to a more productive workout. If you burn some fat at 25 minutes, you will burn more at 45 minutes. The longer you perform a

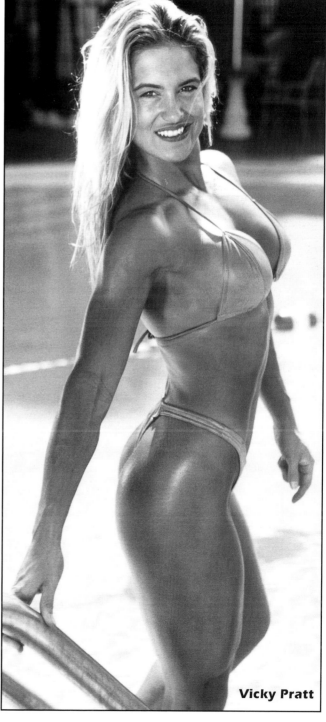

Vicky Pratt

cardiovascular exercise, the more your body burns fat for fuel *after* you have stopped exercising. This is another key principle: The longer the aerobic exercise, the longer the after-workout activity of burning fat for fuel. So make an effort to always extend your aerobic workouts well beyond the 20-minute mark to reap the benefits of having the body burn off that fat.

Nonstop and Semi-hot

There are a couple of other final items that must be factored in to the mix to make the aerobic exercise hit its intended target of using fat for fuel. The aerobic exercise must be continuous (stop-and-rest exercise such as weightlifting is anaerobic and tends to use glycogen instead of fat for fuel) and the exercise must be challenging enough to get the body going at a rate that will burn off fat. In order to successfully

burn fat without going into an overtrained state the heartbeat rate needs to be elevated to between 65 and 85 percent of its maximum heart rate (MHR) during the time that you are training.

Porter Cottrell mentioned 70 percent as the target rate. Others believe that 65 percent is the minimum level for burning bodyfat. You can take the heartbeat rate higher, but the risk is that if you regularly get your heart rate too high, you will quickly put your body into an overtrained state. A long-distance runner wants to elevate his or her heartbeat rate to 85 percent of maximum. If you are trying to also build muscle tone, you don't want to get your heart rate this high. The long-distance runner wants to use the aerobic workout at the upper end of the MHR training range to build endurance, while those whose primary aim is to burn fat while building overall muscle tone will want to use the aerobic workout at the lower end of the MHR training range. A woman who wants to positively reconfigure her physique wants her aerobic exercise to be "semi-hot" – challenging, without going overboard. If you go too hard with your aerobic exercise, you will soon step into the overtraining range and start to become too lean, losing muscle tissue, looking too skinny and emaciated. You want progression, not digression, from your workout. The recuperation system starts to bog down and you won't get the muscle tone

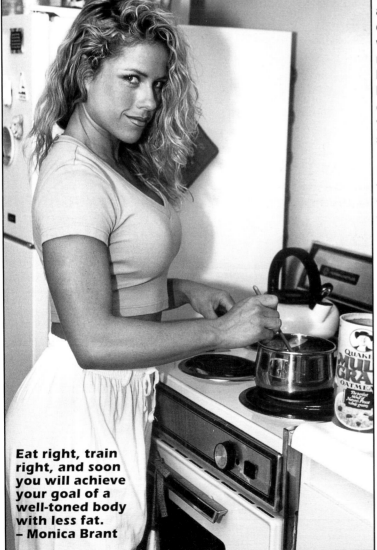

Eat right, train right, and soon you will achieve your goal of a well-toned body with less fat.
– Monica Brant

In order for an aerobic exercise to successfully use fat for fuel, it needs to involve more than 20 minutes of nonstop activity.

The best training zone for aerobic exercise for those trying to burn fat and build muscle tone is at a rate of 65 to 70 percent of maximum heartbeat rate.

that you desire if you push yourself too far. It is crucial to stay within the right training range to maintain good muscle tone while causing the fat to disappear. Cory Everson points out that beginners and those out of condition should aim at a heart rate of 60 to 65 percent; intermediates should aim at 65 to 70 percent; and those advanced in working their physiques should aim at 70 to 80 percent of maximum heart rate. [14]

Since it is important to stay within a certain range to burn bodyfat, it is also important to find your training range. A simple formula will work. Take your age and deduct it from 220. If you are 35, then you would deduct 35 from 220. Multiply

For an aerobic exercise to be truly effective, it must be nonstop and challenging enough to the body.

this number by 65 or 70 percent. This number *(e.g.: 185 x 65 percent = 120; 185 x 70 percent = 130)* is your target heartbeat rate for your aerobic training. You can find your training rate during exercise by taking your pulse for 10 seconds. Multiply this by six (to arrive at one minute) and you will have your current heartbeat rate. You can check it whenever you want. It is a good idea to occasionally check your heart rate to know what level of activity you are functioning at.

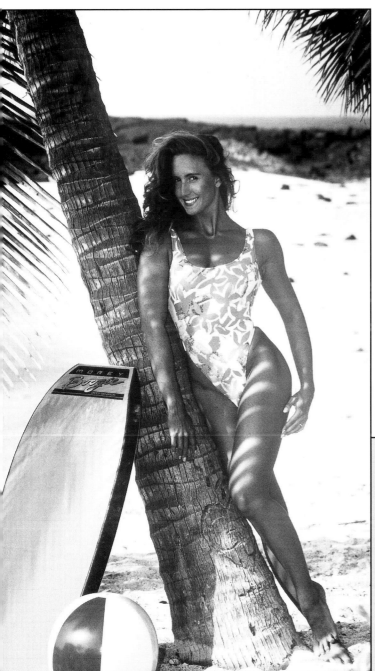

Mo Switzer shows the result of pushing aerobic workouts past the 20-minute mark.

Best MHR Training Zone for Reshaping the Physique:

AGE	65 PERCENT	70 PERCENT
20	130	140
25	127	137
30	124	133
35	120	130
40	117	126
45	114	123
50	111	119
55	107	116
60	104	112
65	101	109
70	98	105

Don't just go to the 20-minute mark with your aerobic exercise; go beyond the 20-minute mark to burn fat.

This range will work well for getting into a training zone to use fat as fuel as long as the aerobic exercise is nonstop work, and lasts for longer than 20 minutes per session.

Frequency

How often should aerobic exercises be performed? Some fitness trainers say that at least three workouts per week are needed. However, even one workout a week is better than none. If you cannot get in three aerobic workouts per week, at least get in one or two per week. The equation is fairly simple – the more aerobic exercises done per week, the more rapid the fat loss. And, of course, these aerobic workouts are qualified according to the guidelines previously provided.

Supercharged Fat Burner

Supercharge your fat-burning by taking an aerobic workout beyond 60 minutes. Research has shown that when the exercise lasts longer than one hour the metabolism stays high and hot for quite some time after the exercise is over, burning off fat long after you have stopped working. Mia Finnegan, winner of the 1995 Fitness Olympia, used 1 1/2 hours of aerobic training a day in preparation for the contest.[15] Of course she was aiming at a title, and you do not want to use this shock effect too

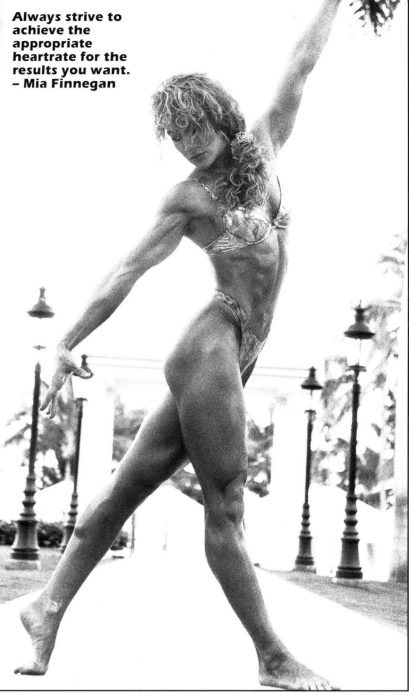

Always strive to achieve the appropriate heartrate for the results you want. – Mia Finnegan

The longer the aerobic exercise session, the longer the after-activity fat-burning effect and the more fat calories that are consumed.

The more aerobic workouts per week, the quicker the loss of bodyfat.

often (to avoid the overtraining syndrome previously mentioned).

Fat for Fuel

Beating fat, getting rid of that unwanted body-weight, is not an easy job – it takes a strong effort and a powerful will to overcome this tenacious body trouble. And it takes something more – the triple combination of diet and the right types of aerobic and muscular exercises. Some people try to win the war over fat with diet alone, but that is not enough. More effort is needed. That effort comes from exercise, but not just any exercise. The exercise needs to be aerobic exercise. It is aerobic exercise that causes the body to burn fat for fuel. Further, a precise type of aerobic exercise is needed to burn off the unwanted fat without taking the body into an overtrained state or causing injury.

The next chapters will focus on the best of the best aerobic exercises that use fat for fuel and allow the muscles to stay well-toned.

References

1. Susan Daniel, "Muscle Media 2000 Index," *Muscle Media 2000* (February 1996), 92.
2. Sergio Oliveira, "Remembrances of a Steroid Gangster," *Muscle Media 2000* (February. 1996), 156.
3. G. Kerry Knowlton, "Bodybuilding BS, Part 1," *Hardgainer* (Jan.-Feb. 1994), 16.
4. Rachel McLish and Joyce Vedral, *Perfect Parts* (New York: Warner Books), 1987, 3.
5. *Walking and Running, The Complete Guide* (Alexandria: Time-Life Books, 1989), 61.
6. Walking and Running, 63.
7. Porter Cottrell, "How to Gain 10 Pounds of Muscle," *Muscle & Fitness* (October 1994), 144.
8. Ruth Silverman, "Fitness Profile: Marla Duncan," *Ironman* (October 1994), 129.
9. Cameo Kneuer, "Anyone Can Have Great Abs," *Muscle & Fitness* (October 1994), 111.
10. "Fitness Profile: Tatiana Anderson," *Muscle Media 2000* (September 1995), 89.
11. Dayna Albrecht, "What To Do After Baby," *MuscleMag International* (April 1995), 184.
12. Nikki Fuller, "Survival of the Fittest," *Flex* (January 1993), 176.
13. Lisa Smith, "Hard Bodz," *Muscular Development* (December 1995), 223.
14. Cory Everson, "Cory's Corner," *Muscle & Fitness* (November 1996), 176.
15. Mia Finnegan and Les Maness, "How I Won The Fitness Olympia," *Muscle & Fitness* (January 1996), 96.

Take advantage of the supercharger effect by adding an occasional workout that lasts for more than 60 minutes.

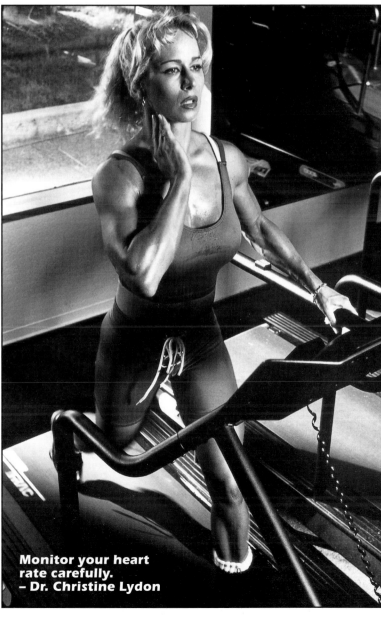

Monitor your heart rate carefully.
– Dr. Christine Lydon

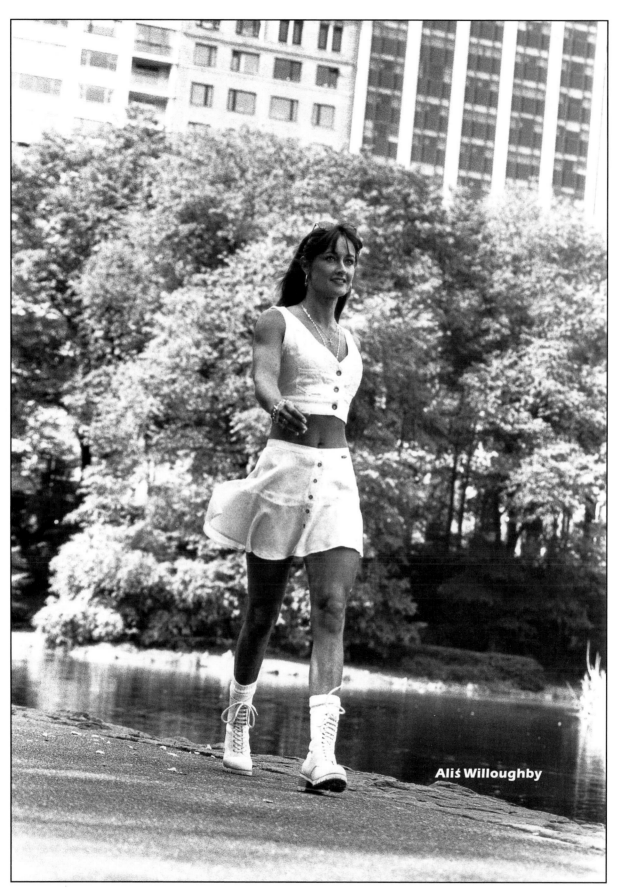

Aliś Willoughby

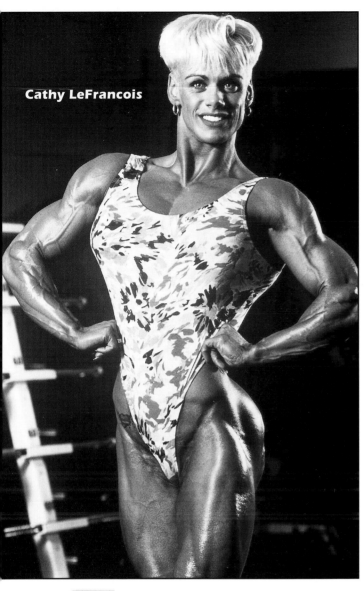

Cathy LeFrancois

CHAPTER TWO

Power Walking – Perfect Exercise for the Physique

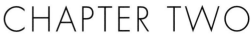

There are literally dozens and dozens of different aerobic exercises that can be performed to work on the physique. From jumping rope to running to rowing, a large array of different exercises produce aerobic results. And it seems that each exercise gets its turn in the spotlight. Running, biking, aerobics, stair stepping, the Nordic track – have all enjoyed center stage of the fitness revolution at some point. And people use many of these exercises to achieve what they want. For example, Tatiana Anderson uses the treadmill, bike, StairMaster, in-line skating, or taking the dogs for a jog for aerobic conditioning.[1] There are dozens of choices for exercises. It can be confusing to try and figure out which exercise to use for aerobic work. But it is important to find an aerobic exercise that will produce the results you want. As mentioned in the last chapter, not all aerobic exercises

work equally well for reshaping the physique. Some aerobic exercises, if used frequently, tend to cut into the muscle tone and shape of the body, or are more likely to promote injuries. And that is just what the person who is interested in reshaping the body wants to avoid – down time due to injury. Fitness star Marjo Selin warns against trying to do too much and overtraining.[2] Tonya Knight points out that certain exercises such as running can cause physical problems and overtraining.[3] When certain aerobic exercises are used on a regular basis, overtraining soon results causing a loss of muscle tone and shape, and certain lower-limb injuries also become a factor, taking away from precious training time. But even considering these problems, aerobic work should not be overlooked or avoided. The right type of aerobic/cardiovascular work can really assist, and is one of the best tools, for cutting off unwanted bodyfat and creating an awesome appearance. Consider what Charles Glass, world-champion physique competitor and one of the top physique trainers around (his clients include such people as Sharon Bruneau, Sylvester Stallone and Wesley Snipes) has to say about aerobic/cardio training: "I have discovered that one of the most crucial

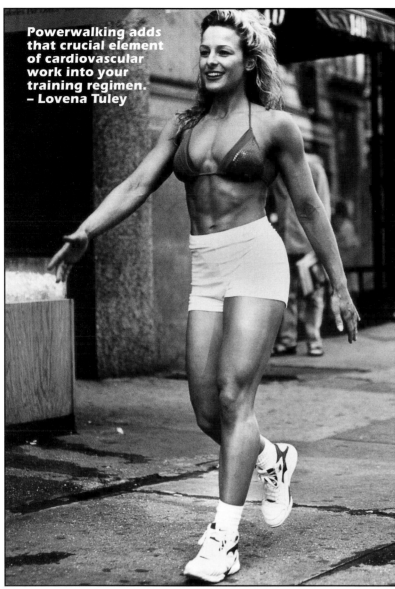

Powerwalking adds that crucial element of cardiovascular work into your training regimen.
– Lovena Tuley

siderations of reshaping the physique are factored in to the aerobic equation, there is one aerobic exercise that stands out far above the crowd for those who want to reshape their body – power walking. Power walking is the "top gun" of the aerobic world when it comes to meeting the unique needs of precisely reshaping the physique. Tonya Knight notes that certain exercises such as running have a negative effect for shaping the physique and she recommends something better – power walking.[6] Power walking is an awesome tool for shaping the physique!

One exercise stands out as the best for reshaping the physique – power walking.

Dynamic Combination

Power walking is the perfect aerobic exercise for reshaping the body. And many people are starting to discover the excellent benefits of power walking. An editor of a natural bodybuilding magazine (who is also a successful competitive bodybuilder) recently ran an editorial where he singled out the fantastic benefits of walking, noting a study that pointed out it was the number one exercise for burning off fat. He is not the only fitness authority to sing the praises of walking. Porter Cottrell uses power walking to stay in superlean condition while maintaining plenty of muscle size and shape. He points out that this walking works in a perfect manner for stripping off fat while leaving the muscle shape.[7] And that is exactly what the body needs – an exercise that strips off unwanted fat while leaving the desirable muscle

elements in training is cardiovascular work. Cardiovascular work, if you are doing it right, really drops the bodyfat for you."[4] Glass goes on to point out that the right type of cardiovascular work really burns the fat off but keeps the muscle.[5]

Not all aerobic exercises work equally well for reshaping the physique.

Top Gun

It is obvious that a woman needs to do aerobic work both for fat loss and health factors – the key is finding and performing the right kind of aerobic work. When all of the various con-

shape. This is not an easy combination for any aerobic exercise to do – but power walking provides it. Power walking, when used on a consistent basis and used for a long enough period, will burn off bodyfat and not burn up muscle tissue in the process. And power walking provides this dynamic combination better than the other aerobic exercises.

The best aerobic exercise for shaping the body is one which strips off the fat while leaving the muscle tone and shape intact. Power walking best fits this requirement.

Power

Power walking must be done with power – hence the name. A Sunday afternoon stroll will not do – you really have to get after it when you power walk. Porter Cottrell says that when he walks, he goes "at a very fast pace, as fast as my legs will take me."[8] This is a very good description of power walking – walking at a pace that is as fast as you can go without breaking into a run. And you do not need to "race-walk" either, where the funny-looking Olympic race-walker stride is utilized. For the shaping of the physique, a regular walk at a fast pace will do the trick. This fast pace walking is similar to marching at a strong clip. (How many fat drill sergeants have you seen? These superfit instructors march most everywhere, and they are supertrim!) Walking can be either aerobic or nonaerobic – it is the pace and

length of the walk that will make the important difference and will make walking work as the fat-burning tool you need.

Power walking is walking at a pace that is as quick as your legs can take you.

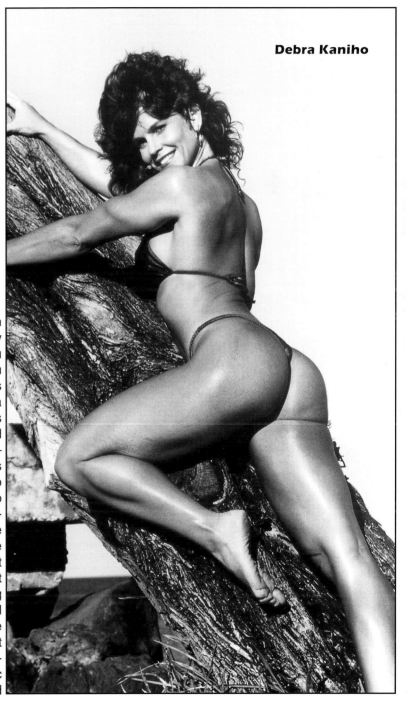

Debra Kaniho

Pace

The pace that corresponds to moving as quick as you can generally falls in the 3.5 to 5 m.p.h. range. Porter Cottrell's speed for his power walking is 2-1/2 miles in 35 minutes. That equates to about 4-1/4 miles per hour. That is a fairly fast rate and a good rate at which to power walk. This rate will elevate the heart sufficiently and burn fat as fuel for the effort. Cameo Kneuer points out that walking should be done briskly. Moving slower than 3 miles per hour will probably not elevate the heart sufficiently and also not use as much fat for fuel.[9]

A good power walking pace to utilize is from 3.5 to 5 miles per hour, on a consistent basis.

Not everyone can start out power walking at an impressive rate. Just as with any exercise, power walking is a progressive endeavor. Practice does not make perfect power walking, but practice does improve the rate at which you move along. Power walking is not the same as running and different muscles are used. As you consistently use power walking your pace will get stronger.

How do you find your individual power walking pace? It is fairly easy to do. Go to a local high school's track, and walk for 30 minutes nonstop at as good a clip as you can manage. Most tracks are a quarter mile in length. Count how many laps you can make in the 30 minutes. For example, if you get around the track 8 times in 30 minutes, then you have covered 2 miles in half an hour. Your speed would be 4 miles per hour (16 laps in 60 minutes). Whatever number of laps you make in 30 minutes is doubled (to arrive at your per-hour rate) and this gives you your rate of speed. Another way to find out your rate of speed is to use a long flat area at which you have noted the mile increments. The track, however, is probably the best way to check your speed since you can be more

Check your pace at a local track once in a while.

exact on the track. Make certain to use the inside lane; the outer lanes cause you to go further than 1 mile per 4 laps (that is why they stagger the lanes for the races). A watch is also a necessity for accuracy in measuring your walking pace.

Once you have your pace for power walking you can walk wherever you want and roughly know how far you have traveled. If you find that you move at a power-walking pace of 4 miles per hour, and you walk for 45 minutes, then you know you have traveled 3 miles. Hills and rugged terrain can cut into your speed, but you still burn as many

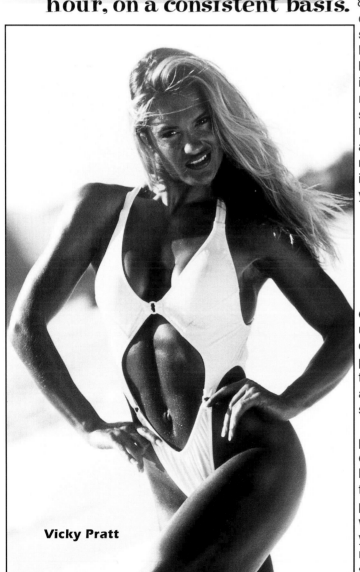

Vicky Pratt

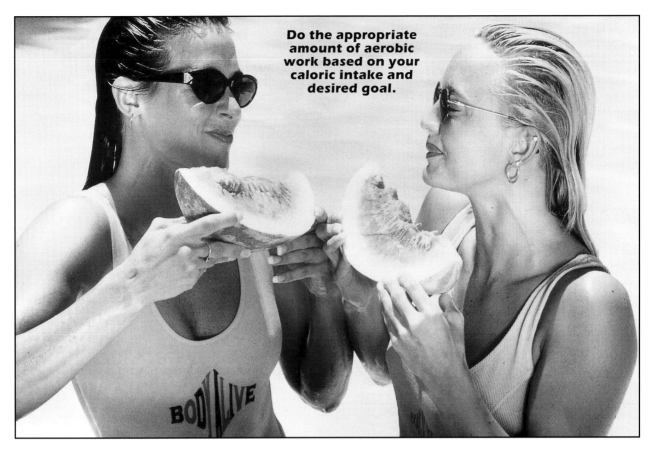

Do the appropriate amount of aerobic work based on your caloric intake and desired goal.

The body starts to burn fat for fuel after about 20 minutes of nonstop aerobic work.

calories or more because of the increased difficulty in body motion. Check your pace once every few months to stay current with your speed.

Duration

How long should your power walk last? You will need to power walk for more than 20 minutes nonstop per workout. The 20-minute mark is the minimum mark for aerobic/cardio work. It is at the 20-minute mark where the body starts to burn fat for fuel, so you want to go beyond 20 minutes to burn off a significant amount of fat. A quick 15-minute aerobic workout is not going to do much for you in burning off fat. The 20-minute mark is a point you should regularly exceed. Of course you may need to work up to going beyond the 20-minute mark initially, but once you have a

Try to get in at least 2 or 3 power walks per week.

few aerobic power walks under your belt you can make a longer walk part of your normal agenda. Power walking at least 30 to 45 minutes per workout is a good target.

If possible, power walk at least twice a week, and preferably more. Cameo Kneuer suggests going for at least three 20- to 30-minute workouts as a minimum per week.[10] If you can get in 3 to 5 power walks per week your bodyfat level should drop noticeably. Physique star Rene Redden performs some type of cardio fitness six times a week and she favors walking.[11] The

The best results come from aerobic exercise performed right after rising or directly after weight training.

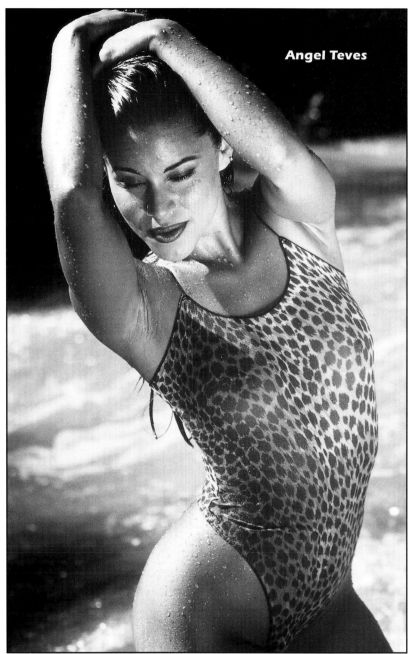

Angel Teves

An occasional 60-minute power walk will really assist in burning off body fat.

great way to take full advantage of your training time and the fat-burning level that your body has attained. Since your body is already hyped up from the weight training it will immediately begin burning fat and will burn fat for the full duration of the power walk. An early-morning power walk works very well also. When you get up in the morning your glycogen storage is low so you tend to more readily burn fat for fuel and an early-morning power walk takes advantage of this, burning a good amount of fat, especially if you go for 40 minutes or more. Cardio, when done on an empty stomach, is the best way to turn up the heat. This will get your metabolism going and get your body to burn up its fat stores.[13] So try to set your aerobic power walking sessions up after lifting weights or upon rising in the morning to maximize the effects and quickly shed fat. You can get that "superfit" look quicker by taking these principles into account.

Power-walking Supercharger

One manner in which to really increase your fat-burning efforts is with the "supercharged" aerobic workout. The typical aerobic workout (which lasts for 30 to 45 minutes) burns off fat as fuel, but research has shown that aerobic workouts that go beyond the 60-minute mark

more you power walk, the more quickly your fat level will decrease.

Time

The best time to perform the power walk is right after getting up in the morning, or directly after a weight-training workout. For supertrainer Charles Glass, the aerobic work comes after the weightlifting session. He gets in 30 to 40 minutes of aerobic training a day, and it always comes after weight training because "at that time, your body is prepared to burn fat."[12] Going for a power walk after a weight workout is a

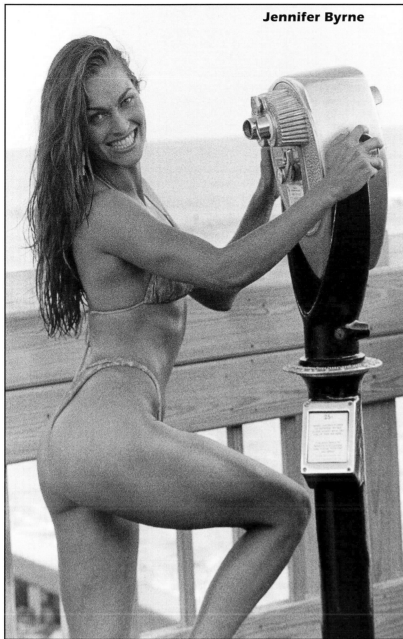

Jennifer Byrne

Consider making power walking the cornerstone of your aerobic exercise program.

Perfect Tool

Power walking is the perfect exercise tool for the woman who wants to burn off bodyfat and still maintain that nice shape of muscle tone. People often search high and wide for some extra training advantage, some special secret to get a handle on their physique and to finally get that "superhot" shape. One of the very best "extra advantages" for getting into lean condition and still having good muscle tone and shape is power walking. When it comes to aerobic exercises that burn off bodyfat, power walking is definitely the best tool to use. Power walking seems to have been designed especially for those interested in reshaping the physique. Regular use of power walking can significantly assist in achieving the unique goals of more muscle tone and shape and less bodyfat. Take advantage of the benefits that power walking provides and use this excellent aerobic tool to cut off that unwanted bodyfat and burn it for fuel.

References

1. "Fitness Profiles: Tatiana Anderson," *Muscle Media 2000* (September 1995), 89.
2. Repping with Marjo, *MuscleMag Intl.* (August 1994), 220.
3. Knight Time, *MuscleMag International* (February 1990), 123.
4. Carol Ann Weber, "Star Trainer Charles Glass Shines," *Muscular Development* (March 1996), 159.
5. Weber, Star Trainer Charles Glass, 159.
6. Knight Time, 123.
7. Porter Cottrell, "How To Gain..," *Muscle & Fitness* (Ocober. 1994), 183-186.
8. Cottrell, "How To Gain…," 183-186
9. Cameo Kneuer, "Anyone Can Have Great Abs," *Muscle & Fitness* (October 1994), 111.
10. Kneuer, Great Abs, 111.
11. Ruth Silverman, "Fitness Profile: Rene Redden," *Ironman* (February 1996), 73.
12. Weber, "Star Trainer Charles Glass," 159.
13. Knight Time, *MuscleMag Intl.* (June 1994), 272.

burn a larger amount of fat and these longer workouts hype the metabolism to such a point that the body continues to burn fat long after the exercise has ceased. The astute woman can take advantage of this factor by going on an extended power walk which lasts for 60 minutes or more. This long power walk will burn off a ton of unwanted fat. It can be performed every once in a while to get the metabolic process burning more fat.

Is power walking the missing tool from your physique-training mix?

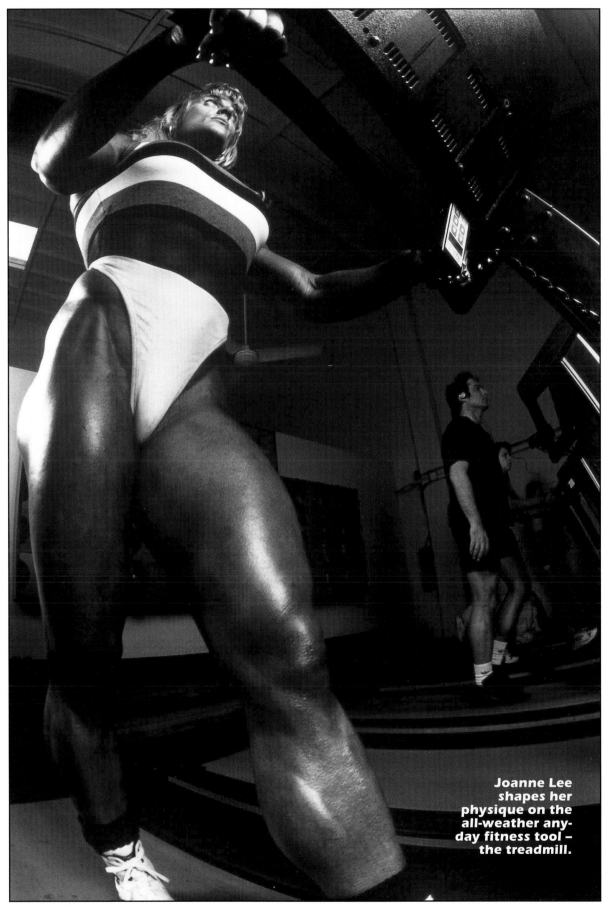

Joanne Lee shapes her physique on the all-weather any-day fitness tool – the treadmill.

CHAPTER THREE

The Terrific Treadmill

Power walking is, without doubt, a fantastic tool for shaping the physique – cutting off bodyfat without cutting into the muscle tone and shape of the body. Power walking on a regular basis really assists a person in achieving the "fitness" look. There is a variation of the power walk that also works well for the fitness approach, and may be even better due to the fact that it can be done in all kinds of weather, and nasty dogs don't chase you when you perform it. This excellent variation of the power walk is the treadmill. The treadmill very effectively uses fat for fuel, perhaps better (for the overall physique-shaping aims) than anything else. Several studies have indicated that fast walking on the treadmill (on a slight incline) is one of the very best ways to burn off a tremendous amount of calories. The treadmill is found in most gyms, and you can buy one at a reasonable price for home use if you want your own. The key features to look for in a good home treadmill are that it is sturdy (frame and treadmill), that it provides sufficient resistance (with a heavy flywheel) and that it is long enough to cover your full stride (some cheap models are too short). It is always best to check one out with these points in mind before purchasing it.

A good treadmill is an excellent home gym tool to use to burn off bodyfat while maintaining a high degree of muscle tone and shape.

The treadmill is effective because, like the regular power walk, it allows you to get in a strong aerobic workout without going too overboard and cutting into muscle tissue or causing injury to your body. And the treadmill does its job of burning off bodyfat (and retaining muscle

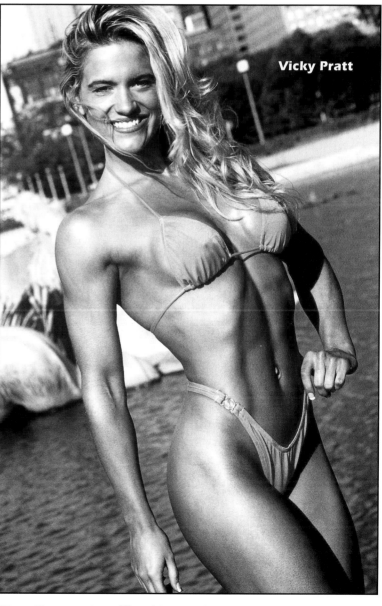

Vicky Pratt

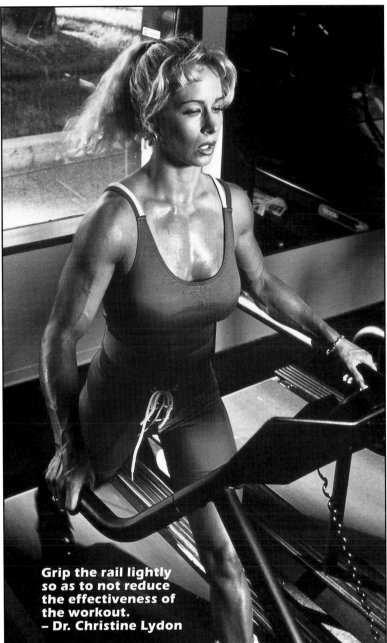

Grip the rail lightly so as to not reduce the effectiveness of the workout.
– Dr. Christine Lydon

Walking on a moderate incline greatly increases the amount of fat calories that are burned off.

Angle

One of the keys to making the treadmill effective for using fat for fuel is to position it at an upward angle when you walk on it. This slight uphill incline is fantastic for burning off even more calories. By using the moderate incline you effectively double the amount of fat calories you are burning off your body as compared to regular brisk walking. Brisk walking on a treadmill at a moderate incline burns off more fat calories than does fast cycling or light jogging.[2] If you are planning on buying a treadmill or using one at the gym, make certain to use or buy one with incline capabilities. Fortunately, most treadmills on the market have this feature.

Progress

Don't immediately start with an incline workout or a long workout. Take a couple of aerobic treadmill workouts at a flat level, then move on to the incline approach. As with any type of fitness endeavor, gradually work up to an increasingly difficult level. Do not start with a hard 60-minute workout. Gradually progress up to the longer time period. Once you are able to go for 30 to 45 minutes you will be at a good range for burning off a portion of fat. Occasionally go for a longer treadmill walk and stay on the machine for 60 minutes or more. This will really increase the amount of fat that is used for fuel, and help your body look better quicker.

Posture

Good posture is important when walking on a treadmill. Do not slouch over or bend your spine. Use a fairly straight-up stance. And don't use the rails to take all your weight off your feet.

tone and shape) very effectively. Charles Glass points out "if you walk that treadmill on an angle at a moderate rate it really burns the fat off but keeps the muscle." Glass walks on the treadmill for 30 to 40 minutes a day, after lifting weights.[1] Many fitness gyms and spas contain a few treadmills so it is easy and efficient for most people to jump on a treadmill after the weight-lifting workout and burn off a lot of extra fat by walking for a few miles. Most hotels and motels also have a fitness room and many have treadmills so you can get in a good aerobic exercise while you are on the road.

A sports doctor advises those who use stair climbers (and this also applies to treadmill use) to hold the rails lightly rather than bracing yourself on them.[3] If you brace yourself on the rails this reduces the effectiveness of the workout. Maintain good posture throughout the walk on the treadmill and let your lower body do most of the work.

Cadence

When working on a treadmill, pick a fairly strong pace. Get your heart rate up to approximately 65 to 70 percent of its maximum. Keep a strong, steady pace, and occasionally move a little faster for variety. Breathe at a steady pace, and have a towel accessible, if possible. You can really sweat while working on a treadmill! Remember to not use the frame for too much support (though some support may be necessary) as this can reduce the amount of calories that you burn.

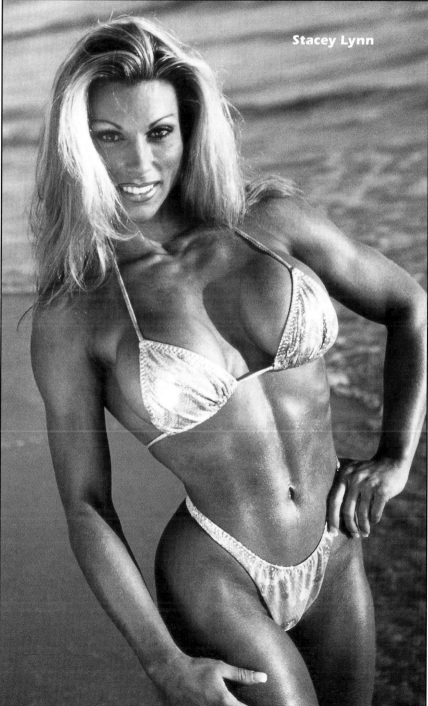

Stacey Lynn

A 45-minute walk on the treadmill is a good level to maintain.

Getting Going

For your first couple of workouts on the treadmill, walk for 15 to 20 minutes. Try to get these workouts in right after weight training or early in the morning. Maintain a strong and steady pace throughout the walk. Once you have this mastered, move up to a 30-minute walk. After you have become used to the 30-minute walk increase your treadmill time to 35 minutes, and then to 40 minutes. After you have gotten a few 40-minute workouts under your belt you can then move on to a 45-minute workout. This is a good level to attain. Aim at being able to handle a consistent 45-minute walk (at a strong pace) on the treadmill. You can even work up to longer levels if you wish, but a strong 45-minute walk on the treadmill will work for most everyone.

Use the treadmill (inside) or power walking (outside) as the foundation for your aerobic work.

Once you have built your stamina up to handle a significant length of time on the treadmill, you can burn even more calories by increasing the angle of the treadmill. The steeper the incline, the more calories you will burn. But as with the time factor, ease into the angle adjustment, moving gradually from a flat plane to a steeper angle. The combination of a steep angle and a strong pace will really burn off significant amounts of bodyfat.

Frequency and Variety

Get in at least two treadmill workouts a week (preferably after a weight-training workout or upon rising) and more if possible. If you can get in 4 to 6 treadmill workouts per week you should rapidly drop your bodyfat composition and start noticing a real "ripped" look. Use the several advantages of the treadmill to get very trim.

Every aerobic workout does not have to be performed on the treadmill – mix different aerobic exercises during the week. This approach alleviates boredom. For example, walk one day, ride the stationary bike on another, and use the treadmill on yet a different day. However, no matter what other aerobic exercises you choose, it is a good idea to use the treadmill as the main pillar of your aerobic exercise structure.

Why use the treadmill as the main aerobic exercise? The treadmill is an awesome tool for stripping off bodyfat and revealing the great muscle tone and shape you have developed. The treadmill is one of the top ways to burn off those ugly fat layers. A recent study involving 13 young, fit volunteers showed that using a treadmill burned more calories than using five other exercise machines. Researchers from Milwaukee's Medical College of Wisconsin and the Veterans Affairs Medical Center found that exercising on a treadmill at a somewhat high level of effort burned 705 calories an hour compared with 627 on the stair machine; 606 on the rower; 595 on the cross-country ski machine; 509 on a stationary bike with handlebars that require a pushing and pulling motion; and 498 on a regular stationary bike.[4]

As you can see, the treadmill is the most productive manner in which to burn off bodyfat in the aerobic exercise arena. When you combine this with the other elements – that it does not tend to cause injury or throw the body into an overtrained state – the treadmill is a great exercise for reshaping the physique. Try the treadmill and find out why it is such a fantastic tool for burning fat for fuel.

References

1. Weber, "Star Trainer Charles Glass," 159.
2. Robert Sweetgall, *Fitness Walking* (New York: Perigee Books, 1985), 159.
3. "Stairway to Fitness," *Muscle & Fitness* (October 1996), 25.
4. *Reader's Digest* (September 1996), 136.

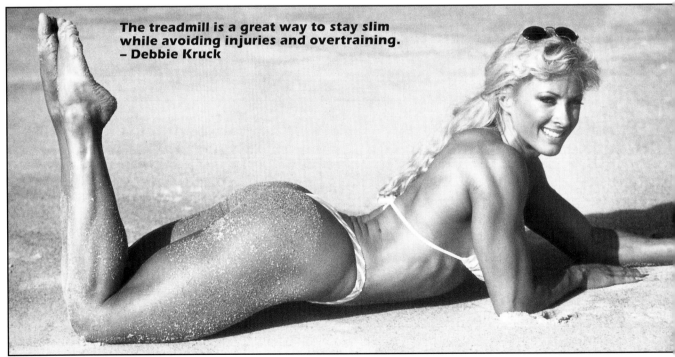

The treadmill is a great way to stay slim while avoiding injuries and overtraining.
– Debbie Kruck

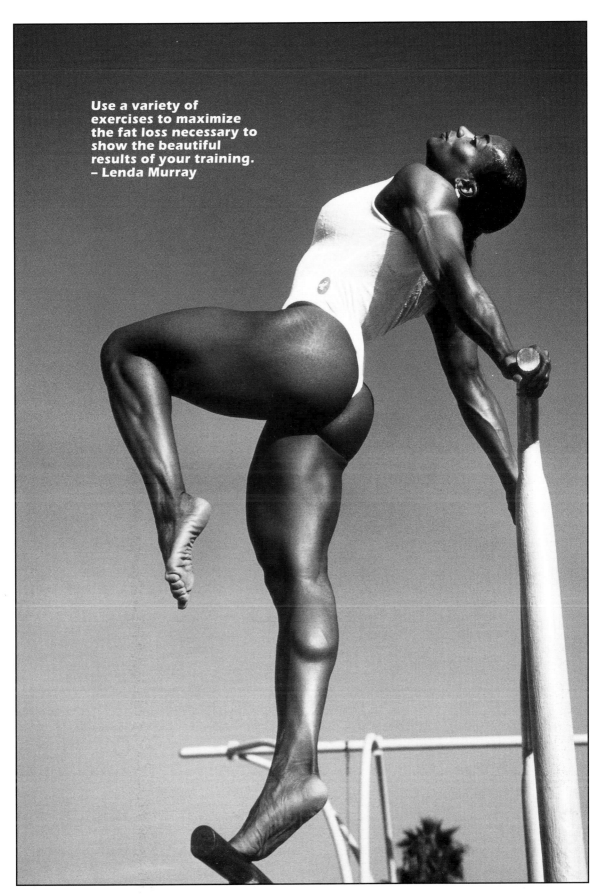

Use a variety of exercises to maximize the fat loss necessary to show the beautiful results of your training.
– Lenda Murray

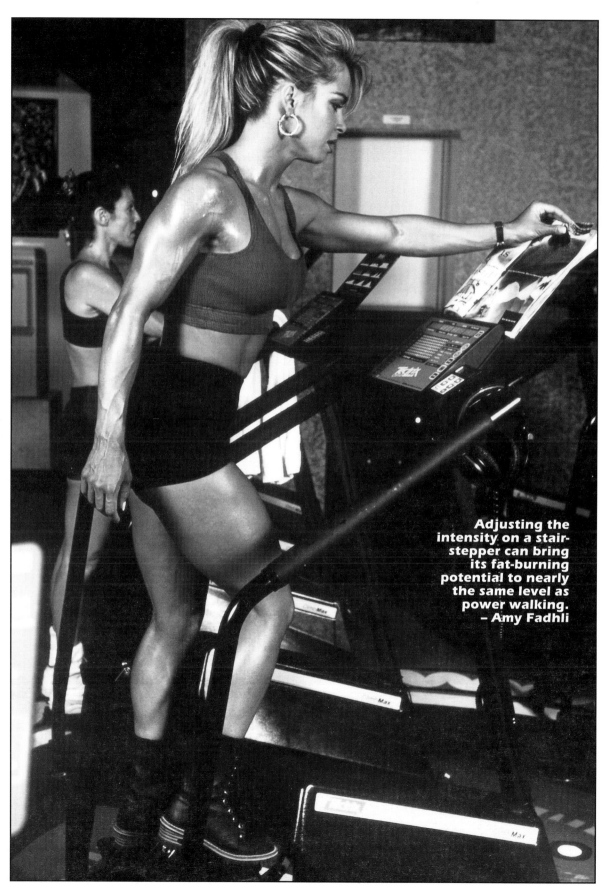

Adjusting the intensity on a stair-stepper can bring its fat-burning potential to nearly the same level as power walking.
– Amy Fadhli

Power walking and fast walking on the treadmill are great exercises, and probably the very best for shaping the physique, when combined with a weight-training program. However, power walking and using the treadmill are not the only exercises that use fat for fuel.

Another exercise comes in a close second for burning off bodyfat and maintaining excellent muscle tone and shape. This excellent exercise is the stair-stepper machine. Research has shown that fast walking on the treadmill will burn 705 calories per hour, and that using a stair-stepper will burn 627 calories an hour. The two exercises also have other similarities. The stair-stepper produces minimal injury risk, and it also does not throw the body into an overtrained state as do some other

aerobic exercises. If you want to build a complete physique, with a combination of leanness, shape and firm muscle tone, and to look like a Marla Duncan, Monica Brant, Amy Fadhli, or Brandi Carrier, then you will need to use an exercise routine that burns off fat while helping to reshape your physique. The stair-stepper is excellent for this purpose.

The stair-stepping machine is also one of the best aerobic exercises for shaping the physique.

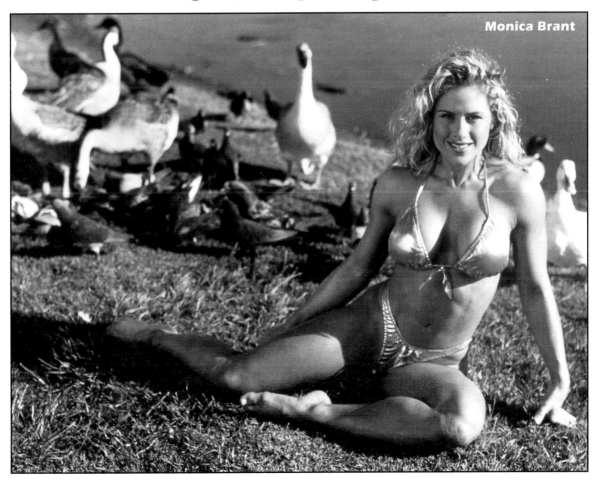

Monica Brant

Using the stair machine causes the body to burn off over 600 calories per hour.

Readily Available

The stair-stepper is a handy exercise because most gyms have several of them readily available. This allows you the opportunity to go directly from a weight-training workout to a fat-burning session on the stair-stepper. You can also perform the stair-stepping exercise at home if you have a personal unit. Stair machines are becoming fairly inexpensive (especially when they go on sale) and you can pick up a used one at a real bargain by checking the newspaper ads. Make certain that the stair machine you purchase (if you choose to go this route) provides a sufficient challenge and is adjustable. There are even very small stair-stepping units available for use while traveling that work well.

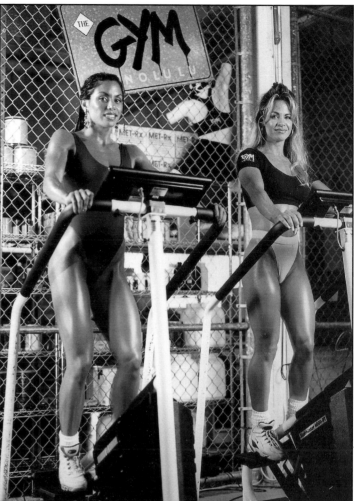

Ursula Alberto and Amy Fadhli burn fat on the stairclimbers.

Real Stair Stepping

There is no law that says you have to perform all of your stair stepping on a machine. And any and all stair stepping is good for you.

One way to lose weight is to stay out of the elevator and off the escalator. Walking up stairs burns 150 percent more calories than playing tennis and 23 percent more than running, reports a Cleveland Clinic study. Just adding two flights of stairs to your normal physical activity each day could lead to a weight loss of 12 pounds in one year.[1]

So take the stairs whenever you have the option of using them. If you live in a mid- to large-sized city, you will probably have the opportunity to use the stairs on a frequent basis.

Any and all stair climbing is great for your physique.

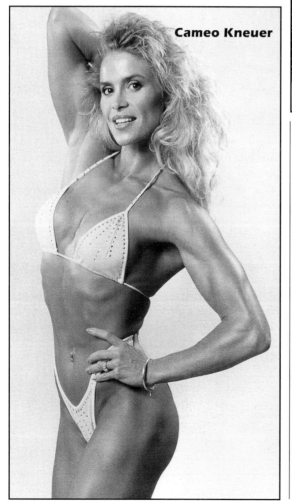

Cameo Kneuer

Aim for a 30- to 45-minute stair-climbing workout, but occasionally go for a longer time period.

Stair climbing is one of the quickest ways available to get rid of fat. And you can get in a fat-for-fuel workout away from the gym at no cost. Climbing stairs in a high-rise building is a great way to burn off fat, and there is an added benefit – it builds great looking legs. One physique professional in particular was noted for using stair climbing in a tall building to build a fantastic and famous pair of legs. So can you. Stair climbing can add some new firm contours to your legs while also burning off bodyfat.

Working Out

Start with a moderate stair-climbing effort, either on the stair machine or on a staircase. Go for 15 to 20 minutes or so to get used to climbing stairs (it can be tough initially, especially if you have not done it before). Gradually work your way up to longer and longer workouts. And remember, once you get used to stair climbing, go beyond the 20-minute mark to make certain that you are burning off fat. Aim at a 30- to 45-minute stair-climbing session per workout, and try to get in a 60-minute stair workout once a month. This will help accelerate your fat loss without cutting into your muscular reserves. A stair-climbing workout after a weight workout is a good way to burn off excess fat, and so is a stair-climbing routine early in the morning.

Rotation

Stair climbing does not need to be performed at every scheduled aerobic session. Rotate the stair-climbing workouts with various other aerobic workouts. Use a couple of stair-climbing workouts mixed in with some treadmill or power walking during the week. Stair climbing does not have to be the sole aerobic exercise you use – vary your aerobic exercise scheme. For instance, Cameo Kneuer alternates the stair-stepper with the treadmill and stationary biking.[2] Nikki Fuller rotates the stair-stepper with other exercises such as swimming, power walking and more.[3] Alternate to prevent boredom.

Stair Climbing

Stair climbing is one of the best exercises for shaping the physique since it allows the body to shed fat without becoming "skin and bones." Add it to your arsenal of effective aerobic exercises and burn fat for fuel by using the stair machine and the stairs on a regular basis.

References
1. Hotline Weight Loss, *Muscle & Fitness* (October 1996), 30.
2. Cameo Kneuer, "Anyone Can Have Great Abs," *Muscle & Fitness* (October 1994), 111.
3. Nikki Fuller, "Survival of the Fullest," *Flex* (January 1993), 176.

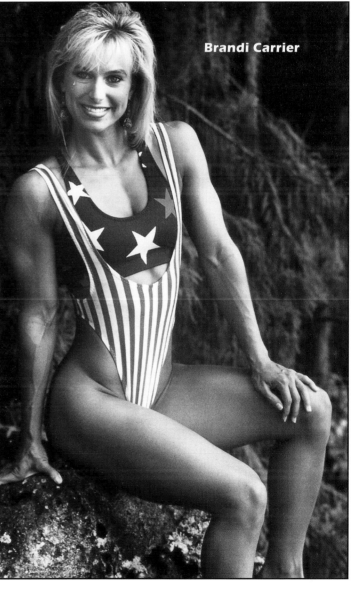

Brandi Carrier

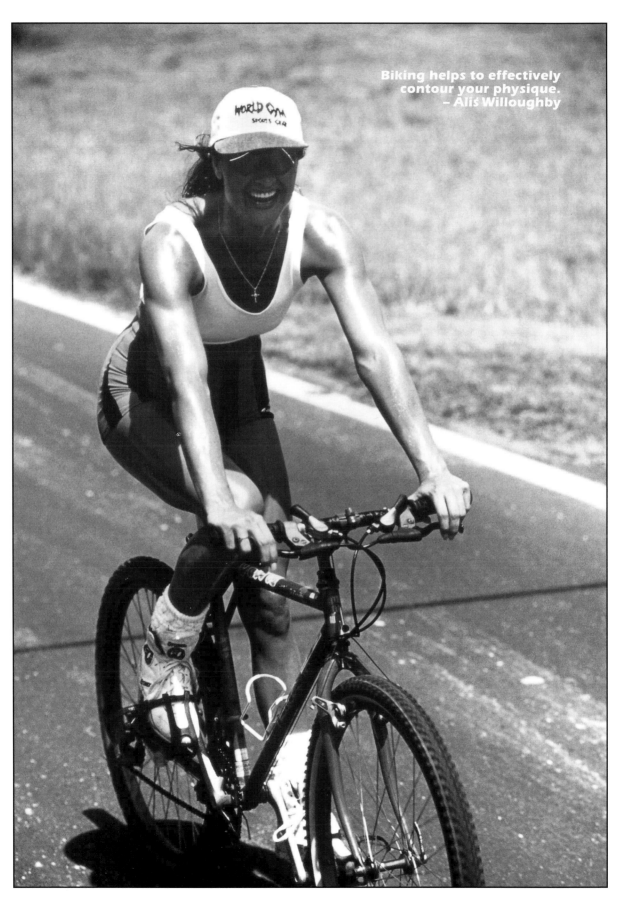

Biking helps to effectively contour your physique.
– Alis Willoughby

CHAPTER FIVE

Burning Off Fat With Biking

Biking is yet another excellent aerobic exercise that works well for body shaping (tone and muscle contours) and burning fat. This popular exercise also has the important combination of burning off bodyfat while not using muscle tissue for fuel, the aerobic combination that is essential for looking great. Biking is one of the better exercises for burning fat for fuel and many physique stars use biking to effectively contour their physiques to just the right dimensions. As with the treadmill and the stair machine, a stationary bike is a common exercise tool that is readily available in most gyms. In fact, most gyms usually have quite a few stationary bikes. And if you want your own, a stationary bike can be picked up fairly cheap for home use when sporting goods stores have sales, or in the ad section of the newspaper. The best stationary bike is one that has a good solid flywheel (for adequate resistance), a timer attached, and wheels that don't squeak.

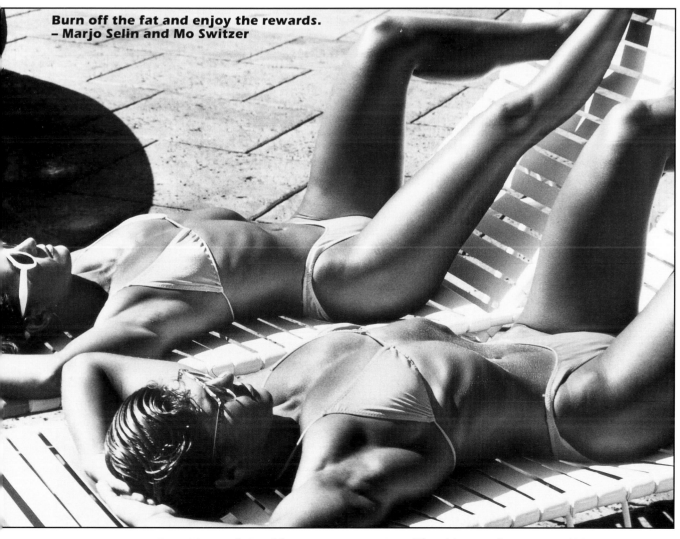

**Burn off the fat and enjoy the rewards.
– Marjo Selin and Mo Switzer**

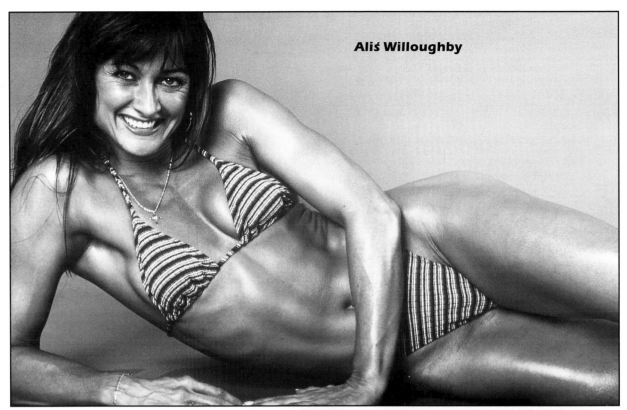

Aliś Willoughby

Use of the stationary bike does not cause the body to burn quite as many calories as does use of the treadmill or stair machine, but the stationary bike still burns a great deal of calories (about 500 calories burned per hour). It, however, taxes the recovery system of the body somewhat less than the treadmill or stair machine, primarily due to the fact that with the treadmill and stair machine the body is in a "weight-bearing" position whereas with the stationary bike the body is supported. You can adjust the resistance of the bike to give you just the right amount of stimulation for getting your body going without taking it too far. It is better

The stationary bike is a nonweight-bearing machine that does not tax the body's recovery system as severely as do many of the other aerobic exercises.

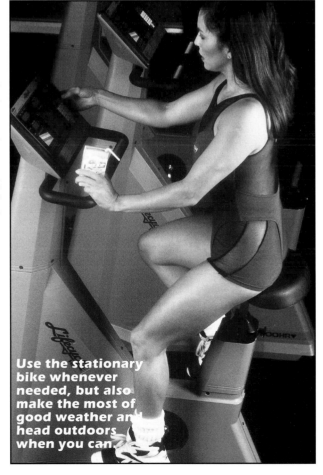

Use the stationary bike whenever needed, but also make the most of good weather and head outdoors when you can.

for body shaping than are certain other exercises, such as running. Tonya Knight points out that "running is not a good aerobic exercise for a bodybuilder because it tears down too much muscle tissue and it is too hard on the joints When running it is very easy to overtrain."[1] Tonya recommends speed walking and stationary biking for aerobic training.

Duration

The minimum amount of time spent on a stationary bike should be at least 20 minutes. A 45-minute stationary bike ride is a good level to aim at, and an occasional longer workout is also a good idea. A stationary bike ride can be taken in the morning before eating or after a weight-training workout for maximum fat-burning effect. Your body is more prone to use fat for fuel at that time. Try to perform several stationary bike workouts during the week, or mix bike riding with power walking, treadmill work, and stair climbing. Those who use the stationary bike often find it to be one of their favorite exercises and continue to use it over a long period of time. Dayna Albrecht rides a bike for 30 minutes daily.[2] Rene Redden, Tatiana Anderson and Cameo Kneuer are others who use the stationary bike to stay in shape.

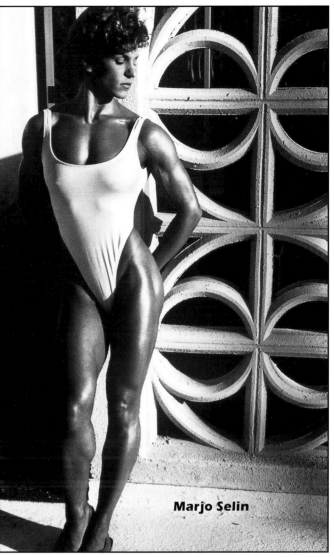

Marjo Selin

The Real Deal

Stationary biking (when used consistently) is a great way to get rid of bodyfat and maintain nice-looking muscle contour, but it is not the only way to get these top benefits. Riding outdoors on a real bike is also a good way to get the same effect and see the scenery to boot. Many prefer to get their biking done in the outside environment if the weather is favorable. Vince Gironda, the super trainer, likes to take a long bike ride on a frequent basis. Many of the photographs in fitness magazines that focus on a fitness star or athlete getting in an aerobic workout feature biking – either stationary or outdoors. Fitness shaping and bike riding go together very well.

The best approach for biking is to use both the stationary bike and the regular bike, varying their use as you desire, and taking advantage of either based on the weather. Having a stationary bike at home is a good idea so that you can get in extra aerobic workouts even on the days that you do not lift weights or go to the gym.

Use biking to burn off bodyfat effectively and maintain muscle tone and shape. Biking is an exercise that uses fat for fuel in a manner that qualifies it as a great exercise for a fitness physique.

References

1. Knight Time, *MuscleMag International* (February 1990), 123.
2. Dayna Albrecht, "What To Do After Baby," *MuscleMag International* (April 1995), 184.

For the best results from biking, mix use of the stationary bike with regular bike rides.

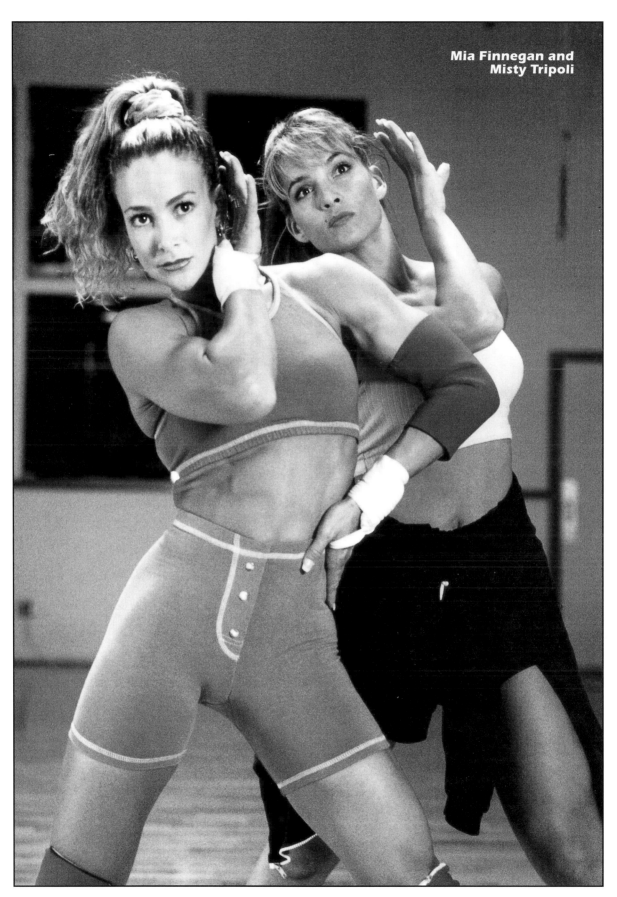

Mia Finnegan and
Misty Tripoli

THE MAGIC OF FAT LOSS – *Lose Fat and Double Your Energy For Life!*

Aerobic describes any type of nonstop movement that burns fat. Power walking, biking, walking on a treadmill, and stair climbing are aerobic exercises. "Aerobics", however, is the name tagged onto exercise that means nonstop full-body motion performed in a certain sequence or rhythmic pattern. Aerobics sessions became quite popular a couple of decades ago, and branched out into such hybrids as "dance aerobics" and "jazz aerobics." Aerobic-style exercise shows are often shown on early-morning television, and can be seen on either regular or cable television. These sessions involve an instructor or two leading a class through certain nonstop movements at a brisk, continuous pace. These aerobics often incorporate dance, military-style free-hand exercises, martial arts moves, calisthenics, stair-stepping, and a variety of other motions.

CHAPTER SIX
Awesome Aerobics

Aerobic-style exercise has several positive advantages. You do not need a lot of fancy and expensive gym equipment to perform aerobics

Aerobics are generally low-impact exercises, with a very minimal chance of injury.

"Aerobics" are a great way to burn off bodyfat and maintain muscle tone and shape.

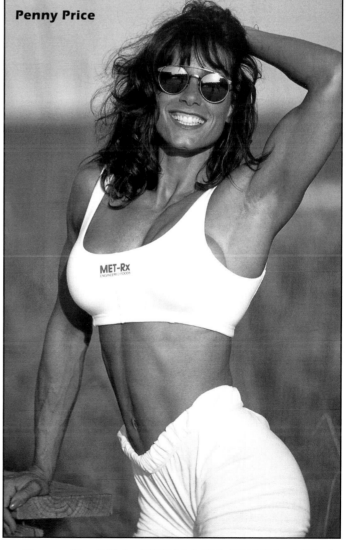

Penny Price

Why are aerobics important? Aerobics are important for the physique simply because these types of workouts, like those mentioned in earlier chapters, effectively burn off bodyfat while leaving the muscle tone and shape intact. Aerobic-style exercises use fat for fuel and do it well. Even guys use them now. "Believe me, a few years ago you would never have caught me dead in an aerobics class," says personal trainer Lawrence Phillips. Now he is a top aerobics instructor. Phillips tells his aerobics class "you're not adding size (by performing the aerobics) but you're not tearing down muscle either. As long as you stay in the fat-burning zone, your muscles will stay nice and toned and lean."[1] As Phillips points out, aerobic-style exercise uses fat for fuel, carving in the curved look.

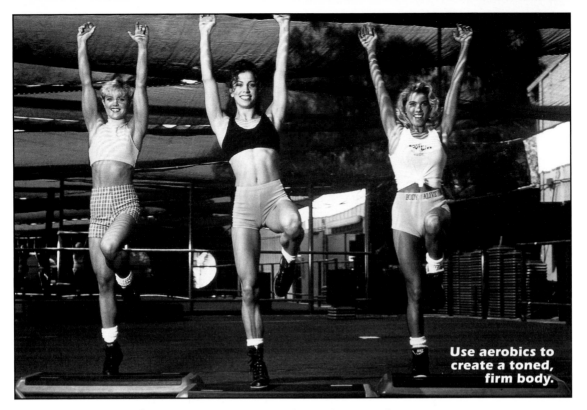

Use aerobics to create a toned, firm body.

Aerobic exercise is not easy.
Nonstop full-body motion can be tough!

– you can get in a great workout without paying a single penny for equipment. You simply move your body in a certain patterned groove. Another benefit is that you can also perform aerobics when you are traveling and don't have access to a fitness facility. If you use aerobics, you can still get in a fat-burning workout in your room. Yet another advantage of aerobics is that they are generally considered to be low-impact exercise. This means they provide a very minimal chance of injury. The movement in aerobics does not involve placing a heavy strain on the body. And as with most all general aerobic exercises (treadmill, stair machine, etc.), aerobics that are performed on a regular basis are good for total-body health, benefitting the heart, lungs and all other body systems.

If you are creative, you can perform your own aerobics routine. If you are not, turn on the television in the morning and watch a couple of the aerobics sessions until you get the idea. Follow the routines for a couple of weeks and you should be able to memorize most of the routine. If you have to, you can buy an aerobics video tape and follow along as the instructor guides you. Otherwise, your own ideas should be sufficient, and cheaper. The main idea is to keep moving nonstop and to get all of the main muscle groups involved at one point.

Slowly increase the length of your aerobics workout. Aerobics is not for sissies and is not as easy as everyone may think. Lawrence Phillips notes that "a lot of bodybuilders and football players come in (to his aerobics class) thinking they can breeze through it. They don't last very long, though."[3] It is difficult initially to move continuously for a long period of time, especially if you have not done so previously. Aerobics keeps you moving and burns off bodyfat. And that is the goal of any good fitness routine. If you want to look hot, like a Penny Price, a Mo Switzer, or a Rachel McLish, you have to burn that fat as fuel. Aerobics is one good way to do so. And if you need accountability in sticking with your aerobics workout, you can always join an aerobics class. Whether in a class or at home, you burn the same amount of fat calories, and that is the goal – using fat for fuel while keeping your muscle tone and shape in fantastic condition. Aerobics works well to achieve this goal. Try them.

References
1. T.C. Luoma, "Get Chizzled or I'll Rip Your Throat Out," *Muscle Media 2000* (July 1995), 43.
2. Luoma, "Get Chiseled or I'll Rip Your Throat Out," 44.

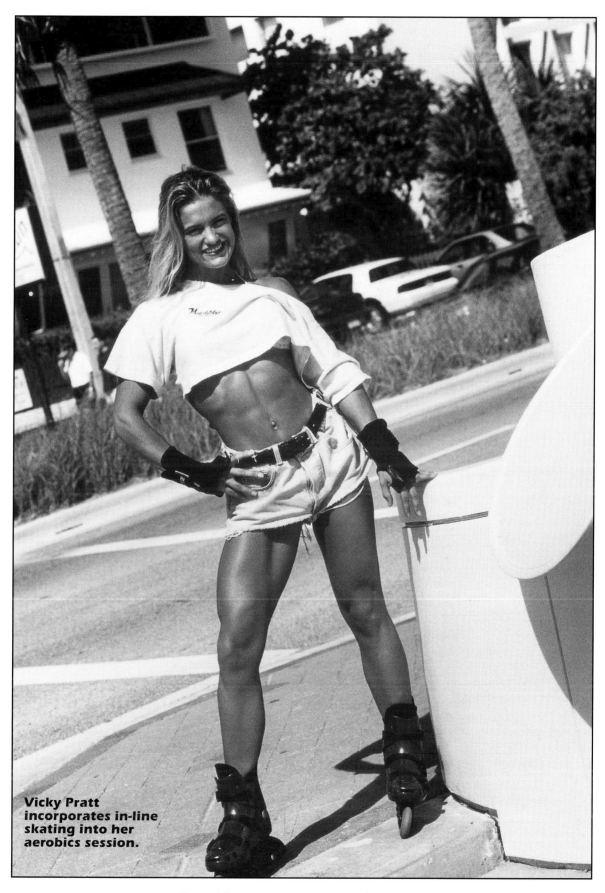

Vicky Pratt incorporates in-line skating into her aerobics session.

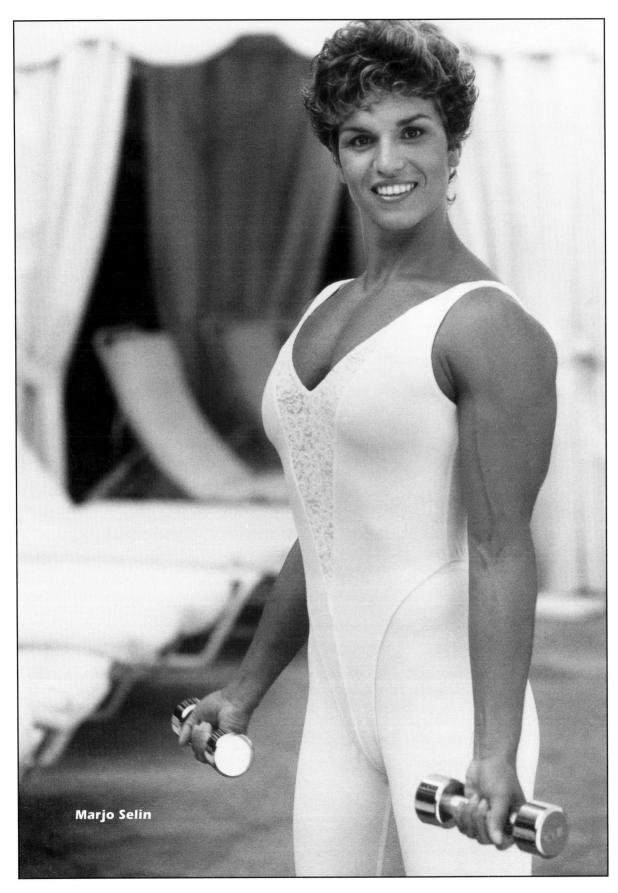

Marjo Selin

Weight training is an activity not usually associated with a fat-burning effect. Most people who are knowledgeable in the area of fitness know that weight training is not an aerobic exercise. It is an anaerobic exercise. As such, it causes the body primarily to burn glucose for fuel instead of fat. But wait, before you toss out weight training, there is good news about it and fat burning. When you weight train, you build up your muscle. And when you have more muscle, you burn more fat, *even as you rest.* The resting metabolic rate of muscle is much higher than that of fat. Muscle, even when it is resting, is still fairly active. So if you have more muscle, you will automatically burn more fat. The key is to add some muscularity to your physique – not a huge amount, but just a nice increase of muscle – so

CHAPTER SEVEN

Weight Training Works Wonders

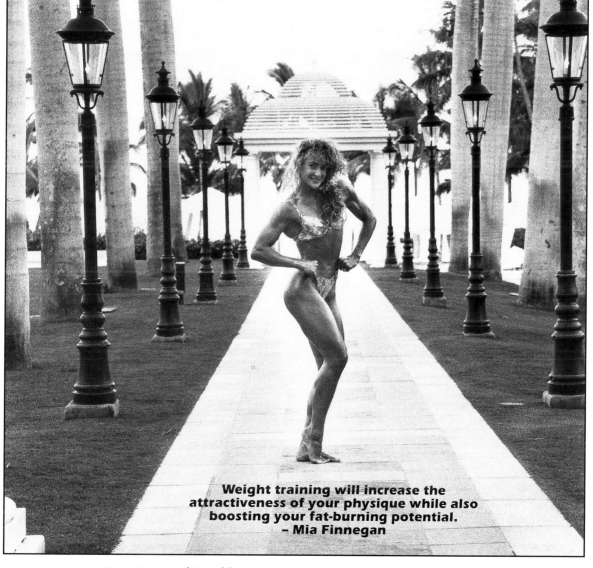

Weight training will increase the attractiveness of your physique while also boosting your fat-burning potential.
– Mia Finnegan

Lose Fat and Double Your Energy For Life! – **THE MAGIC OF FAT LOSS 47**

that you will burn more fat throughout the day. This muscle has the added benefit of increasing the attractiveness of your physique also, making your body firm all over.

More muscle comes from exercise that stimulates the body to increase lean muscle size. Weight training is the superior manner in which to promote muscle growth, shape, and tone. By using weight training on a con-

Weight training is a wonderful way to hype your metabolism to burn off fat on a consistent basis!

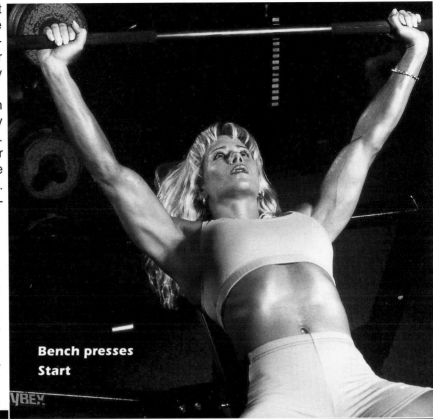

Bench presses
Start

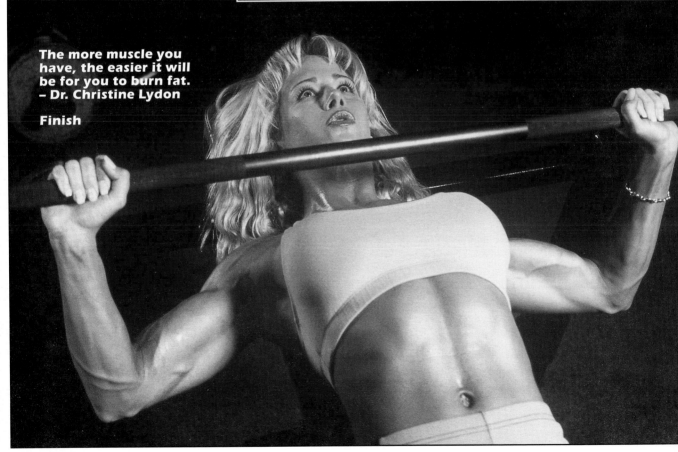

The more muscle you have, the easier it will be for you to burn fat.
– Dr. Christine Lydon

Finish

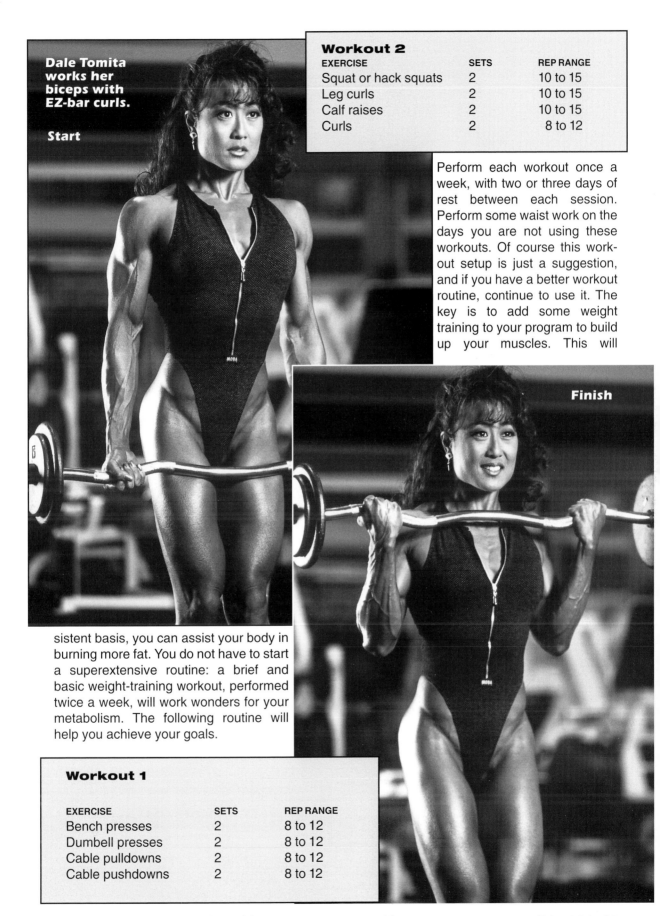

Dale Tomita works her biceps with EZ-bar curls.

Start

Finish

Workout 2

EXERCISE	SETS	REP RANGE
Squat or hack squats	2	10 to 15
Leg curls	2	10 to 15
Calf raises	2	10 to 15
Curls	2	8 to 12

Perform each workout once a week, with two or three days of rest between each session. Perform some waist work on the days you are not using these workouts. Of course this workout setup is just a suggestion, and if you have a better workout routine, continue to use it. The key is to add some weight training to your program to build up your muscles. This will

sistent basis, you can assist your body in burning more fat. You do not have to start a superextensive routine: a brief and basic weight-training workout, performed twice a week, will work wonders for your metabolism. The following routine will help you achieve your goals.

Workout 1

EXERCISE	SETS	REP RANGE
Bench presses	2	8 to 12
Dumbell presses	2	8 to 12
Cable pulldowns	2	8 to 12
Cable pushdowns	2	8 to 12

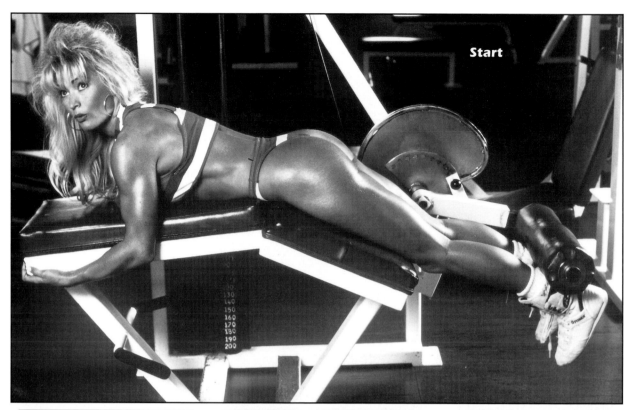

Start

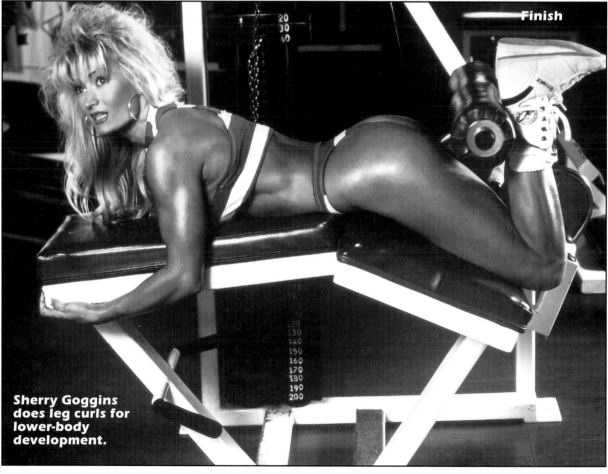

Finish

Sherry Goggins
does leg curls for
lower-body
development.

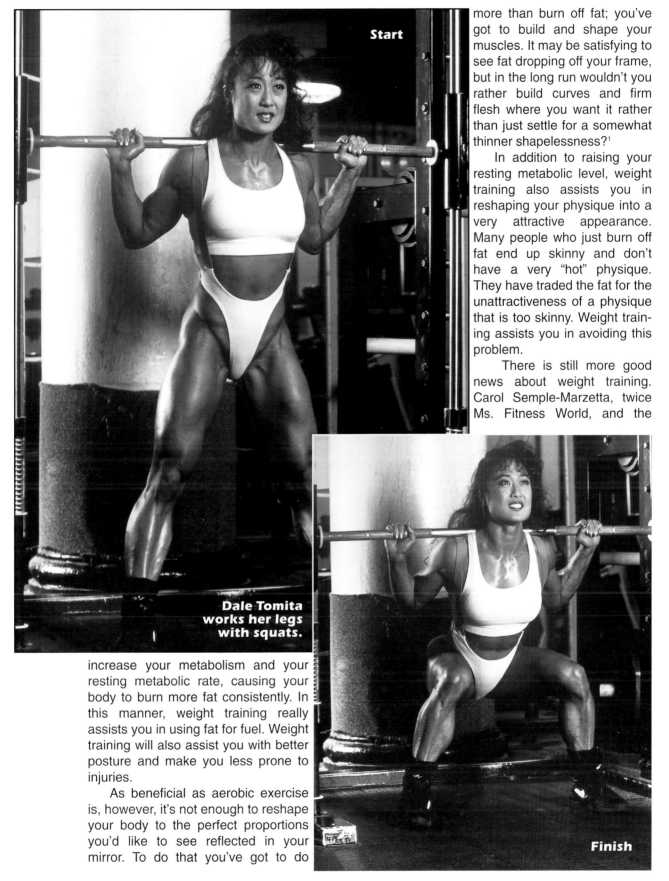

Start

more than burn off fat; you've got to build and shape your muscles. It may be satisfying to see fat dropping off your frame, but in the long run wouldn't you rather build curves and firm flesh where you want it rather than just settle for a somewhat thinner shapelessness?[1]

In addition to raising your resting metabolic level, weight training also assists you in reshaping your physique into a very attractive appearance. Many people who just burn off fat end up skinny and don't have a very "hot" physique. They have traded the fat for the unattractiveness of a physique that is too skinny. Weight training assists you in avoiding this problem.

There is still more good news about weight training. Carol Semple-Marzetta, twice Ms. Fitness World, and the

Dale Tomita works her legs with squats.

increase your metabolism and your resting metabolic rate, causing your body to burn more fat consistently. In this manner, weight training really assists you in using fat for fuel. Weight training will also assist you with better posture and make you less prone to injuries.

As beneficial as aerobic exercise is, however, it's not enough to reshape your body to the perfect proportions you'd like to see reflected in your mirror. To do that you've got to do

Finish

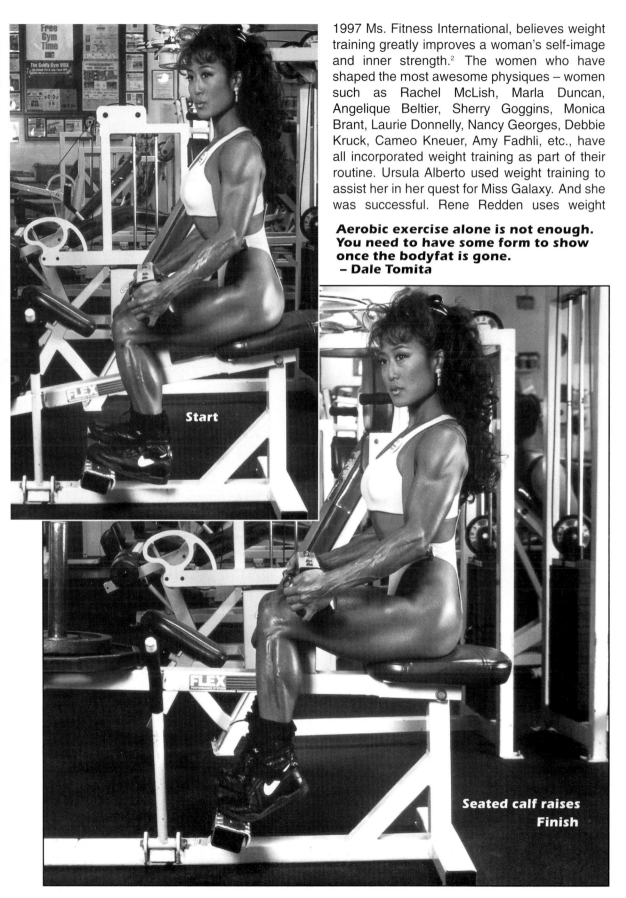

1997 Ms. Fitness International, believes weight training greatly improves a woman's self-image and inner strength.[2] The women who have shaped the most awesome physiques – women such as Rachel McLish, Marla Duncan, Angelique Beltier, Sherry Goggins, Monica Brant, Laurie Donnelly, Nancy Georges, Debbie Kruck, Cameo Kneuer, Amy Fadhli, etc., have all incorporated weight training as part of their routine. Ursula Alberto used weight training to assist her in her quest for Miss Galaxy. And she was successful. Rene Redden uses weight

Aerobic exercise alone is not enough. You need to have some form to show once the bodyfat is gone.
– Dale Tomita

Start

Seated calf raises
Finish

training. So does Dale Tomita. Sharon Bruneau used weight training to change her physique. Wherever you find a lady who has successfully reshaped her physique, you will most likely find that weight training played a part in the transformation.

Take advantage of the many benefits of weight training – particularly to increase your metabolism, reshape your physique, and change the way you look. A weight-trained physique burns fat for fuel and looks great.

References

1. Rachel McLish and Joyce Vedral, *Perfect Parts* (New York: Warner Books, 1987), 3.
2. Michelle Basta Boubion, "Should Women Weight Train Like Men?" *Muscle & Fitness* (November 1996), 80.

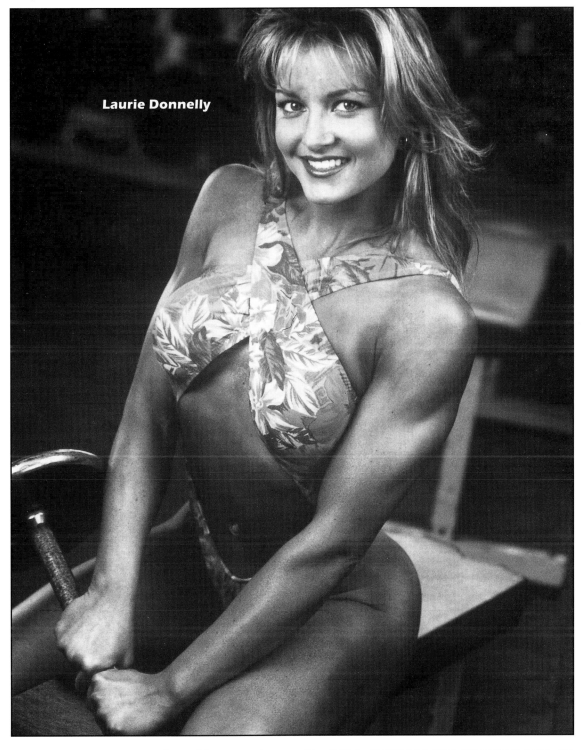

Laurie Donnelly

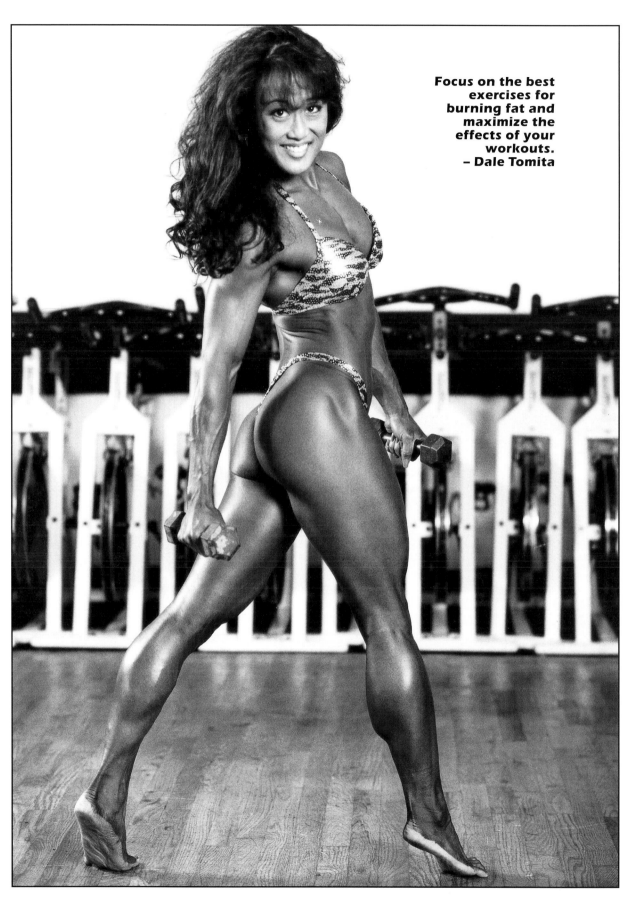

Focus on the best exercises for burning fat and maximize the effects of your workouts.
– Dale Tomita

CHAPTER EIGHT

The Total Mix

The aim of this book is to point out the exercises that are best suited for contouring the body into super shape. Certain aerobic exercises work better than others for providing the combined effect of burning fat for fuel while also working well with the muscle tone and shape of the body. These exercises – power walking, treadmill, stair climbing, stationary bike, and movement aerobics – are the best for what is necessary for reshaping the physique.

When used regularly and for *more than* 20 minutes per workout, these exercises burn off significant amounts of bodyfat. And these exercises don't present the problems for the physique such as injuries and overtraining that other cardio/aerobic exercises do. If you are wise and select one of these choice aerobic exercises to burn fat for fuel, you can start to contour your body into the shape that you want, get rid of fat and reveal a new look. Use of the aerobic exercises advocated in this book can help you avoid the other aerobic exercises that are not as productive (and sometimes negative) for achieving the goals you want. Don't waste time on exercises that do not meet your needs for reshaping your physique – focus on the best exercises, those that use a lot of fat for fuel and keep your muscles toned and well-shaped.

Choose one of the better aerobic exercises – power walking, treadmill, stair-stepping, stationary bike, or motion aerobics – to maximize the benefits of your aerobic training.

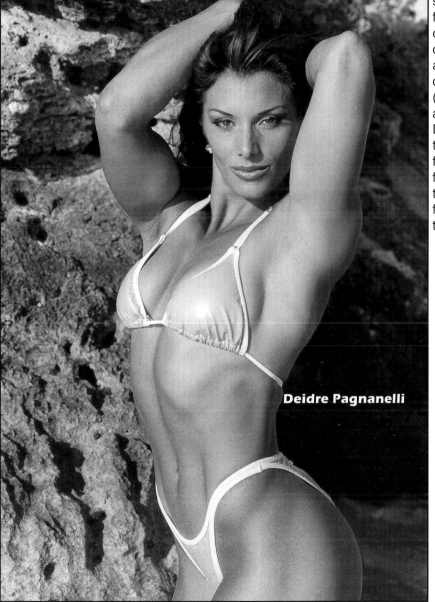

Deidre Pagnanelli

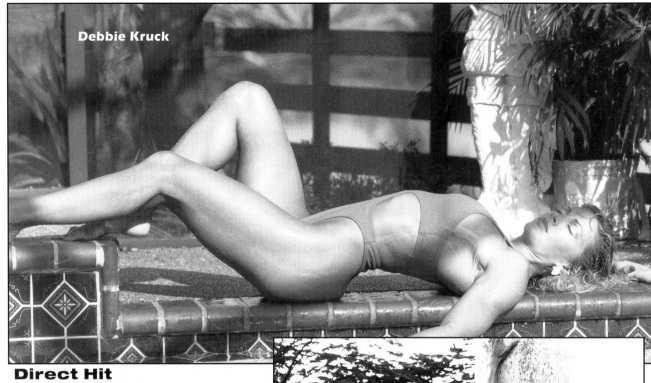
Debbie Kruck

Direct Hit

When choosing an aerobic exercise, don't stumble around with a variety of exercises that are less than the best. Go for a direct hit – an aerobic exercise that is effective in the ways the body needs in order to be re-contoured. Use one of the aerobic exercises listed in this book. Which one? Any of the ones featured in the past chapters will do. Power walking, the treadmill, stair-stepping, riding a bike, and movement aerobics will all help you burn bodyfat. You can use one of these exercises exclusively, or you can rotate with a couple of them. Fitness star Renee Redden uses body-sculpting and step classes, walking, the stationary bike, and the stair machine.[1] She gets a good workout rotation, and alleviates training boredom.

Variety – The Spice of a Continual Routine

You will probably find one of these aerobic exercises is more productive for your needs than the others, but remember that variety is productive for the physique. And variety is not only the spice of life, it can also be the spice that makes an aerobic routine continually effective. You can beat the problem of boredom that often accompanies aerobic workouts by occasionally switching to a different type of aerobic exercise.

Another consideration when it comes to variety is to not totally ignore running, or

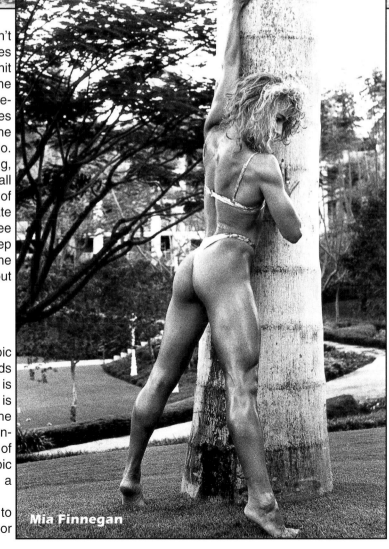
Mia Finnegan

some of the other aerobic exercises. Running, as mentioned earlier, is not the best aerobic exercise for reshaping the body (because if it is performed too frequently or long it can lead to overtraining or injury), but an occasional run will actually be good for the body, as will an occasional use of some of the other aerobic exercises. But make these sessions occasional, and not frequent. If you perform four or five aerobic exercises a week, only run once a week. When you start using an exercise like running too frequently you will most likely find that the results will clash with your physique-shaping goals. So for the most part, stick with the "prime" exercises listed in *The Magic of Fat Loss.*

You can build a body that is more trim, muscular, and contoured. If you use the exercises in *The Magic of Fat Loss* in the manner prescribed, you should notice that you are starting to get that "hot" appearance. Give your diet a hand in the battle against bodyfat – use some of that fat as fuel. And don't forget the benefits of weight training for burning more fat for fuel – particularly in the area of your resting metabolism. And you can further assist your fat-burning program by being more active in general.

Move it or lose it! Walk, climb stairs, stretch, bicycle, dance, play a musical instrument, clean house, watch preschoolers, play with your pet, wash your car, mow your lawn, garden. Be more active in your everyday activities to help burn off fat. Even fidgeting and kissing burn calories.[2] More activity will help you become or stay trim. So get busy and burn fat for your fuel.

References
1. Ruth Silverman, "Fitness Profile: Renee Redden," *Ironman* (February 1996), 73.
2. Everyday Activities, *Muscle & Fitness* (November 1996), 103.

A very healthy and happy Vicky Pratt.

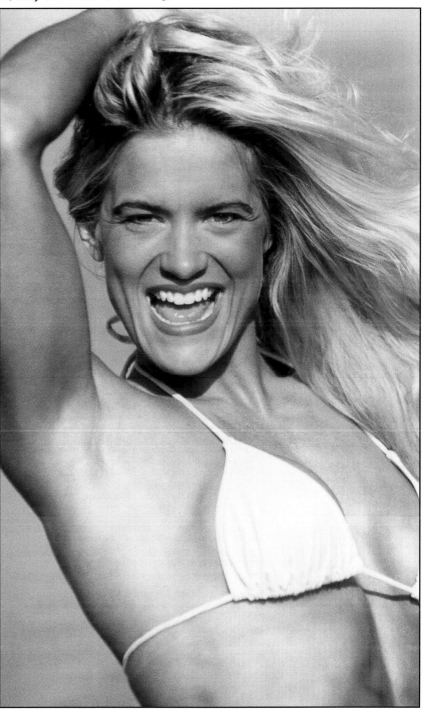

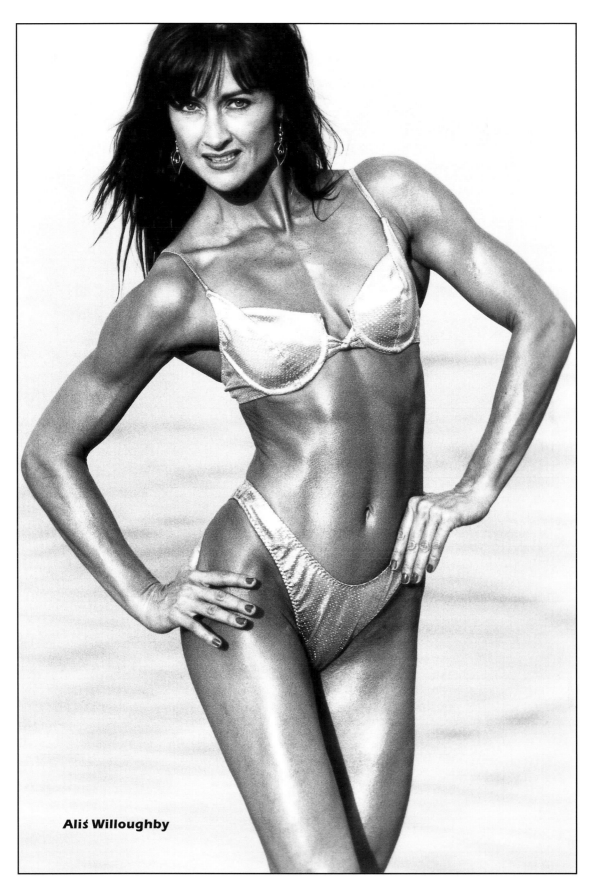

Aliś Willoughby

Index

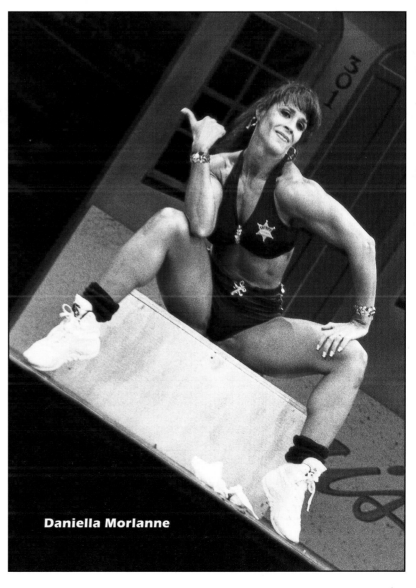

Daniella Morlanne

K

M

P

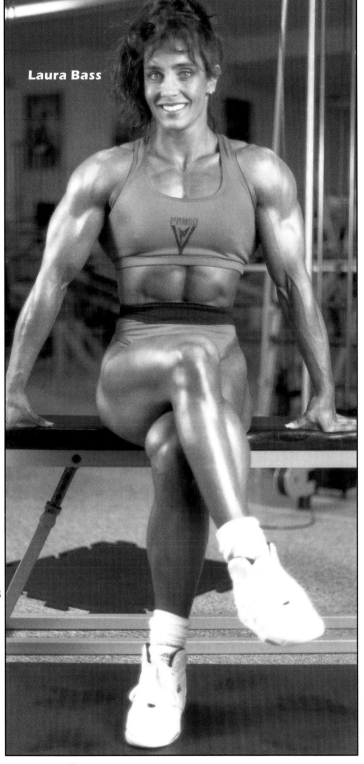

Laura Bass

R

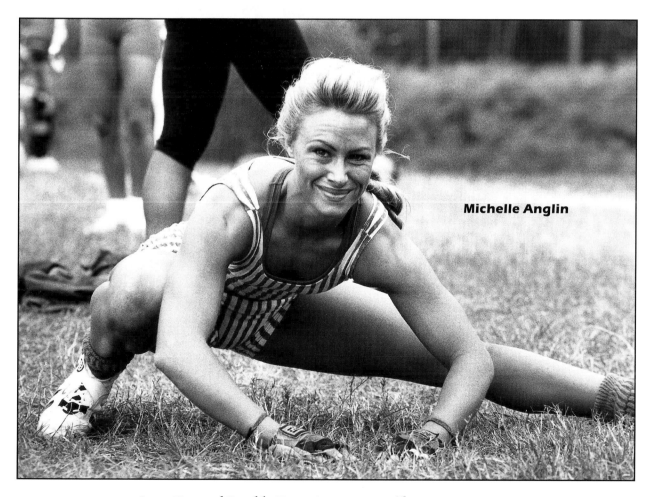

Michelle Anglin

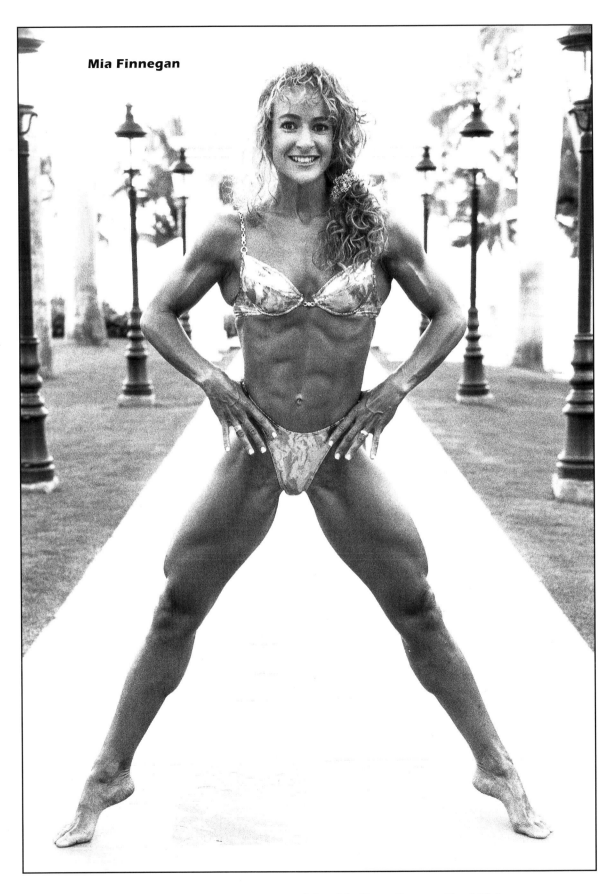

Mia Finnegan

<u>Contributing photographers</u>
Jim Amentler, Alex Ardenti, Doris Barrilleaux,
Garry Bartlett, Reg Bradford, James Cohn,
Paula Crane, Ralph DeHaan, Tony Duffy,
Francis Faulkner, Irvin Gelb, Robert Kennedy,
Marconi, Mitsuru Okabe, Rena Pearl